THE PHYSICAL AND MENTAL HEALTH OF AGED WOMEN

Marie R. Haug, Ph.D., received her doctorate in Sociology from Case Western Reserve University and has been teaching there since 1968. In addition to being Professor Emerita of Sociology, she is also the Director Emerita of the University's Center on Aging and Health. She has published widely, in books and professional journals such as the *Journal of Gerontology,* the *Journal of Health and Social Behavior,* and *Medical Care.* Recent works edited by Dr. Haug include *Elderly Patients and Their Doctors, Depression and Aging: Causes, Care and Consequences,* and *Communications Technology and the Elderly: Issues and Forecasts.* She is also co-author of *Consumerism in Medicine: Challenging Physician Authority.*

Amasa B. Ford, M.D., received his degree from Harvard Medical School and trained in internal medicine at Massachusetts General Hospital and University Hospitals of Cleveland. From 1954 to 1969 he was on the staff of Benjamin Rose Hospital (geriatrics) where he served as Medical Director from 1960 to 1969. He is currently Professor of Epidemiology and Community Health and Family Medicine, Associate Professor of Medicine, and Associate Dean for Geriatric Medicine, at Case Western Reserve University School of Medicine, Cleveland, Ohio. Dr. Ford has done research in heart disease, geriatrics, work physiology, health services, and epidemiological aspects of community health. He is the author of *The Doctor's Perspective* and *Urban Health in America,* and is co-editor of two forthcoming books, *The Practice of Geriatric Medicine* and *Suicide in Children and Adolescents.*

Marian Sheafor, R.N., Ph.D., is currently Associate Dean for the Graduate Program at The Intercollegiate Center for Nursing Education in Spokane, Washington, and Professor of Nursing, Washington State University. At the time this book was prepared, she was a member of the gerontological nursing faculty of Frances Payne Bolton School of Nursing, Case Western Reserve University, and a Senior Faculty Associate of the Center on Aging and Health. Her work has appeared in the *American Journal of Nursing, Nursing Outlook,* and *Geriatric Nursing.*

THE PHYSICAL AND MENTAL HEALTH OF AGED WOMEN

Marie R. Haug, Ph.D.
Amasa B. Ford, M.D.
Marian Sheafor, R.N., Ph.D.

Editors

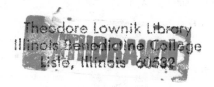

SPRINGER PUBLISHING COMPANY
New York

Copyright © 1985 by Springer Publishing Company, Inc.
All rights reserved

Springer Publishing Company, Inc.
536 Broadway
New York, New York 10012

85 86 87 88 89 / 10 9 8 7 6 5 4 3 2 1

Library of Congress Cataloging in Publication Data

Main entry under title:
The Physical and mental health of aged women.

  Bibliography: p. Includes index.
  1. Aged women–Care and hygiene–United States.   2. Aged women–Medical care–
United States.   3. Aged women–Mental health–United States.   4. Aged women–
Diseases–United States.   5. Aged women–United States–Social conditions.   I. Haug,
Marie R.   II. Ford, Amasa B.   III. Sheafor, Marian.   [DNLM: 1. Aging.   2. Health
Services for the Aged.   3. Mental Health–in old age.   4. Women.   WT 104 P5775]
RA778.P54   1985   362.1'9897   84–26870
ISBN 0-8261-4340-7

Printed in the United States of America

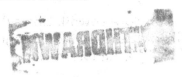

Contents

VI   HEALTH CARE ISSUES   217

Contributors

Faye G. Abdellah, R.N., Ed.D., F.A.A.N. (D.Sc., LL.D., Hon.), Deputy Surgeon General and Chief Nurse Officer, U.S. Public Health Service

Susan Beggs Baker, M.P.H., Ph.D., Assistant Professor of Community Medicine, Baylor College of Medicine

Irene Burnside, R.N., M.S., F.A.A.N., Assistant Professor, Department of Nursing, San Jose State University

Irven DeVore, Ph.D., Professor of Anthropology and Biology, Harvard University

Robert B. Greenblatt, M.D., Professor Emeritus of Endocrinology, Department of Endocrinology, Medical College of Georgia, Augusta

David L. Gutmann, Ph.D., Professor of Psychiatry and Education, Northwestern University Medical School

Gunhild O. Hagestad, Ph.D., Assistant Professor of Human Development, College of Human Development, Pennsylvania State University

Charles E. Holzer III, Ph.D., Assistant Professor of Psychiatry and Sociology, and Depression Research Unit, Department of Psychiatry, Yale University School of Medicine

Charles L. Hoppel, M.D., Department of Medicine, VA Medical Center, Cleveland

Jacquelyne Johnson Jackson, Ph.D., Associate Professor of Medical Sociology, Department of Psychiatry, Duke University Medical Center

Boaz Kahana, Ph.D., Professor and Chair, Department of Psychology, Cleveland State University, Cleveland, Ohio

Eva Kahana, Ph.D., Professor of Sociology and Director, Elderly Care Research Center, Case Western Reserve University, Cleveland, Ohio

Anthony Karpas, M.D., Internal Medicine Group, 478 Peachtree St., N.E., Atlanta

Philip J. Leaf, Ph.D., Assistant Professor, Departments of Psychiatry, Sociology and Institution for Social and Policy Studies, and Depression Research Unit, Department of Psychiatry, Yale University School of Medicine

Robert Lindsay, M.B.Ch.B., Ph.D., M.R.C.P., Professor of Clinical Medicine, College of Physicians and Surgeons, Columbia University; Chief Executive Officer and Director, Regional Bone Center, Helen Hayes Hospital, West Haverstraw, New York

C. Owen Lovejoy, Ph.D., Professor of Anatomy and Anthropology, Kent State University

Carol O. Mitchell, Ph.D., R.D., Assistant Professor of Medicine, Division of Hematology and Oncology, University of Arkansas for Medical Sciences, Little Rock

P.K. Natrajan, M.D., Department of Endocrinology, Medical College of Georgia, Augusta

Matilda White Riley, D.Sc., Associate Director, Behavioral Sciences Research, National Institute on Aging, National Institutes of Health

Anne R. Somers, B.A., D.Sc. (Hon.), Professor, Departments of Environmental and Community Medicine and Family Medicine, University of Medicine and Dentistry of New Jersey-Rutgers Medical School

Carlos Vallbona, M.D., Professor and Chairman of Community Medicine, Professor of Rehabilitation and Family Medicine, Baylor College of Medicine

Lois M. Verbrugge, M.P.H., Ph.D., Associate Research Scientist, Institute of Gerontology; Faculty Associate, Survey Research Center, Institute for Social Research, The University of Michigan

Myrna M. Weissman, Ph.D., Professor of Psychiatry and Epidemiology; Director, Depression Research Unit, Department of Psychiatry, Yale University School of Medicine

Claude E. Welch, M.D., D.Sc. (Hon.), Clinical Professor of Surgery Emeritus, Harvard Medical School; Senior Surgeon, Massachusetts General Hospital

Mary Opal Wolanin, R.N., M.P.A., F.A.A.N., Associate Professor of Nursing Emeritus, University of Arizona

Preface

Whistler's Mother or the Grey Panther's Maggie Kuhn—these two images of elderly women demonstrate how wide a variety of roles they may play in American society. Underlying this diversity, however, are some uniformities. Women's common physical and biological makeup may be one factor in their longevity, currently an average life expectancy exceeding that of males by about five years. Extended life is not necessarily a boon if morbidity, low income, and isolation diminish the quality of the additional years. Nevertheless many women, relying on a store of coping skills acquired over a lifetime, manage their aging very well. Thus the theme of this book is that women may be vulnerable in several ways, but that they can also command strengths to deal with their problems as they age.

There have been various estimates of the size of the future elderly population, depending on assumptions about fertility rates and improvements in disease control. One of the more conservative projections is that by the year 2000 there will be more than 31 million persons aged 65 and above, of whom about 14 million will be at least 75 years old, with the "old-old," those 75 plus, the fastest growing cohorts. Given a continuation of current gender ratios among the elderly, females will constitute 56 percent of those 65 to 74, and 65 percent of those 75 and over. Health professionals will, as a consequence, be required to deal with increasing numbers of elderly women in hospitals, clinics, long-term care institutions, and ambulatory private practice. The need for increased training programs for health care practitioners who deal with the elderly has been underscored by Kane, Solomon, Beck, Keeler, and Kane (1980), without, however, focusing on the unique constellation of health and social needs of old women. Indeed, much of the material on geriatric care fails to take gender differences into account.

Yet professional writing specifically related to old women's health at first appears voluminous. A recent seven-year literature search on the topic of "Health Issues of Older Women" yielded over 950 references. However, approximately two-thirds of these on more careful assessment appeared not to be concerned specifically with the health of older women but merely had some reference to elderly females in their scope. Of the remaining one-third of the citations (about 300), most dealt primarily with issues surrounding menopause. The range of topics discussed in relation to the climacteric period of a woman's life was wide, including the use of hormone replacement therapy, risk of endometrial cancer, and psychosocial and sexual considerations. Thus much of the literature to be found under the heading of "Health Issues of Older Women" actually dealt with middle-aged women—chiefly those under 65 years of age, in their 40s and 50s. An occasional reference to much older women is likely to appear as an individual case history, and some research reports on particular illnesses and conditions did encompass women over 65. Topics covered included osteoporosis, hypochondria, depression and the senile dementias, cancer, incontinence, and mental confusion, among others. Missing, however, is an integrated approach to the health and welfare problems of aged females.

More importantly, the literature tends to overlook the special strengths that could be invoked by old women to cope with these problems. A major purpose of this book is to present just such an integrated approach to the diverse mental, physical, and living problems of elderly women, and at the same time to offer a perspective on their coping abilities.

Accordingly, the book tends to both the vulnerabilities and the strengths of old women, the benefits as well as the costs of gender differences, and in so doing integrates behavioral and medical perspectives on this growing segment of the population. DeVore and Lovejoy show, from the point of view of physical anthropology, that females are not the weaker sex, and even that in some animals males are unnecessary to the perpetuation of a species! Riley warns against the stereotyping of old women by reminding the reader of cohort differences, while Somers describes the demographic revolution being brought about by the growing numbers of elderly, particularly female elderly.

General physical health data on older women as compared to older men are provided by Verbrugge in an epidemiological profile; Greenblatt and colleagues discuss the health relevance of estrogen and the female reproductive system; and Lindsay describes the bone loss that characterizes many women of advanced years. Turning to mental health issues, Gutmann analyzes the stresses and potentials of developmental changes as women age, with Holzer and colleagues showing that depression, despite popular beliefs, is not more prevalent or less treatable among older women than among younger ones. Wolanin approaches the problem of mental confusion from a similar optimistic stance, stressing that its effects can be alleviated and managed.

Health professionals are increasingly aware of the inseparable link between social factors in the lives of their patients and their physical and mental health. The roles of family conflict or cohesion, grief, isolation, and other forms of socially induced stress in producing illness are more and more widely recognized. In this book the social situations that impinge on elderly females are reviewed in terms of both the intimacy of the family and the discriminatory practices found in society. Hagestad explores the effects of intergenerational relationships on aged women, both as positive supports and as sources of conflicts. Burnside focuses specifically on the impact of losses—spouse, children, or pets—on the well-being of the frail elderly. Jackson suggests that aged black women may not suffer from claimed multiple jeopardies, an ill-defined term, since racism is the dominant social fact affecting their lives.

Issues in treatment and care are approached as nutritional, surgical, and pharmacological problems. Selection of these three treatment modalities from among the many that could have been singled out was dictated by their special importance to older women, coupled with their relative neglect in the health literature. For example, women's longevity can lead to isolation, with implications for adequate nutrition, an undervalued health issue. Among the consequences of long life are frailty, falls, and fractures requiring surgery, sometimes unnecessarily viewed as contraindicated at advanced ages. The risk of polypharmacy as a result of the multiple chronic conditions likely among the very old, chiefly women, is not well understood by some practitioners. Mitchell reviews the difficulty in avoiding malnutrition among older women, particularly widows, while Welch describes the possibility of surgical interventions for eight common problems experienced by aged women. The complexities of pharmacological treatment, and their relevance to the physical characteristics of the elderly, are the topics of Hoppel's chapter. Vallbona and Baker review the problems of physical disability in old women and their potential for rehabilitation. Abdellah describes current dilemmas in health care delivery for the old. One aspect of such care, institutionalization, is explored by Kahana and Kahana, who analyze both the problems and positive aspects of the use of long-term-care institutions for aged women.

Finally, in an "Epilogue," the editors review prospects for treatment and research concerning this segment of the elderly population.

By combining behavioral and medical approaches, this book offers health care practitioners, service providers, family members, and aged women themselves cause for optimism about the potential for a positive quality of life for members of the "second sex" in their final years.

M. Haug
A. B. Ford
M. Sheafor

PART I

INTRODUCTION

Three ways of setting the stage for an examination of the strengths and vulnerabilities of aged women are presented in these chapters. Although utilizing widely different perspectives, all three implicitly or explicitly offer evidence of the dangers of stereotyping women, or relying on popular beliefs about their characteristics and roles.

Matilda White Riley, of the National Insitute of Aging, makes as her main theme that aging is not a fixed process, but is subject to social and historical modification. Using the cohort paradigm, she shows how women born during different historical periods have varying educational, marital, work, and health care experiences, as well as being exposed to disparate physical and normative environments. Changes in sex roles, sex ratios, labor force participation, and cigarette smoking have had particularly dramatic effects on cohort characteristics. Women whose life course has been patterned by their membership in different cohorts will exhibit wide variability in their aging. Warning against the fallacy of interpreting age differences in cross-sectional studies as indicating the effects of aging, Dr. Riley, in her highly instructive chapter, notes the implications of rising longevity and technological advances for future elderly women, those now in their early adulthood and middle years. Her chapter is a powerful argument against the easy generalizing that lumps all old women into one category.

Anne Somers' focus on demographic trends supports and expands on Riley's article. The aging of the population, the growing proportion of women among the elderly, and the shrinking of the family are demographic facts that have important consequences for the whole society, and particularly for old women. Some of these consequences include rising health care costs and increasing numbers of old women dependent financially on their own resources, but for whom social security and medicare benefits will be inadequate. A particularly significant issue for the future involves the change in the nature of the electorate, with the emergence of a "female gerontocracy," as younger women, whose views on political issues diverge markedly from those of men in their cohort, reach old age. Dr. Somers concludes with six proposals for the social adjustments needed in order to maintain a creative balance between the concerns of younger and older cohorts.

Physical anthropologists DeVore and Lovejoy make the startling point that males are "an experiment in nature," and perhaps a transitory one at that. Females, far from being the weaker sex, are actually stronger, and in many forms of life do not require another gender for reproductive purposes. In a fascinating review of the question currently engrossing many biologists, "Why are there males at all?," these authors argue that the reason may be efficiency in creating genetic variety. Females also are the basis of most mammalian herds, as well as the fundamental links in the economy of primitive peoples. The critical role of the female in all species destroys the myth of feminine weakness and underscores the reality of women's strengths, both physical and social.

M.H.

1

The Changing
Older Woman:
A Cohort Perspective

MATILDA WHITE RILEY

A recent annual meeting of the Institute of Medicine focused on the goal of postponing the disabilities of old age, of maintaining health and functioning of future cohorts of older people up to the end of the life span. Without diminishing the importance of providing long-term care for the disabled elderly, my goal is to reduce the need for such long-term care, especially for those women who constitute the majority of older people. We all know that some people lead long, healthy, effective, fulfilling lives, while other people succumb early to ill health, unhappiness, loneliness, and withdrawal from affairs. The social and behavioral sciences show that the differing ways in which people age are influenced, not only by biology, but also by the kind of society in which they live—by the work they do, the people they interact with, the households they live in. It has been well documented that aging is a psychosocial, as well as a biomedical, process. Thus I want to remind us of the central proposition that *aging is not an immutable or biologically fixed process, but changes with social structure and social change.* Furthermore, there is an important corollary to this principle: *aging is subject to social as well as medical modification and intervention.*

This interaction between social change and aging processes (both biological and behavioral) can be understood through the cohort approach. I shall discuss three aspects of this approach:

First, the research *paradigm* that underlies it;
Second, *how* social change does indeed influence the aging process, for better for worse;

Third, what can be done to *improve* health and functioning of
women at work, at home, at leisure, by *modifying* both individual lives and the changing social environments that influence these lives.

THE COHORT PARADIGM

I start with a statement of promise. A cohort perspective helps us
to understand the social, psychological, and biological aging processes, as these respond to social changes and can lead to physical
and mental health (or ill health) of aged women today; and it
helps us to understand the potentials for improved health in the
cohorts of women now young who will be old in the future. If
you will lend me your imaginations for a moment I can begin to
fulfill on the promise. I'll do this by sketching a highly abstract
scheme (cf. Riley, 1980).

You can imagine the rough outlines of the paradigm if you
think of a space bounded on its vertical axis by years of age
(from 0 to 100 or so), and on its horizontal axis by historical
time (as from 1900 to 2000 and later). Within this space, think
of a succession of diagonal bars. Each bar represents a cohort of
people—male and female—all born during the same time period.
Within each cohort, people are *aging*—moving across time and
upward with aging. These people as they age change socially and
psychologically as well as biologically; accumulating knowledge,
attitudes, and experiences; moving through social *roles* in family,
school, and work. In the meantime *new cohorts* of people are
continually being born, aging from birth to death, and moving
through historical time. At any single period of history (such as
1982), think of a cross-sectional slice through the successive cohorts that divides people into *age strata,* from the youngest to the
oldest. The people in these strata coexist and are continually interacting with one another. At any given period an epidemic or an
economic depression can cut through all the age strata, impinging
on different cohorts at their respective ages, and affecting the
future course of all their lives and changing their interrelationships
with one another.

This schematic representation is useful because it forces us to
keep in mind that each cohort cuts off a unique segment of historical time—confronts its own particular sequence of social and environmental events and changes. The paradigm brings us inexorably

to the recognition of my central proposition: because society changes, the modal patterns of aging of people in different cohorts cannot be precisely alike (Ryder, 1964). Members of United States cohorts who are old today were born early in this century, grew up prior to the discoveries of antibiotics or the polio vaccine, experienced two World Wars and the Great Depression. These people cannot have aged in precisely the same way as cohorts who lived in earlier times, or as those cohorts now in their younger years who will grow old in the future. At my age my grandmother was certainly no match for me in climbing mountains, working an 18-hour day, or spinning out new paradigms for understanding aging. Nor is it likely that I am any match for my granddaughters when they reach age 70. Aging is mutable, hence subject to social intervention and modification.

SOCIAL CHANGE AND COHORT DIFFERENCES

So far what I have done is to suggest how cohort analysis helps us to link up social change and the aging process. This recognition that people in different cohorts (born at different times) age in different ways has led to research on *how* particular social conditions and changes influence aging—and especially to research on how disability and dependence can be prevented or postponed, how health and functioning can be enhanced across the entire life span (Riley & Bond, 1983). From such research it is now clear that cohorts already old differ markedly from cohorts not yet old in many critical respects: in diet, exercise, standard of living, education, work history, medical care, experience with chronic versus acute diseases. Successive cohorts of young people are on the average taller than their parents, and successive cohorts of young women start to menstruate at younger ages. Let us consider three or four examples of how successive cohorts age in different ways as society changes.

Changes in Sex Roles

A frequently noted change affecting the life course of successive cohorts of women has to do with sex roles and the long-term pressures toward greater equality between men and women. We can see how quickly social change can occur by looking at "Middle-town," that sociological laboratory originally established by Robert and Helen Lynd. Over the last half century, the percentage of Middletowners who felt that homemaking skills were the most desirable attribute for a mother dropped from 57 to 41 among men, and among women, from 52 to 24 (*Behavior Today*, 1979)! Today this new equality is expressed both in the labor force and in new family roles.

A process is at work here which I have elsewhere (Riley, 1978) called "cohort norm formation" (a useful new concept in the cohort approach). That is, many individual women in the cohorts now in their 30s and 40s have responded to common *social* changes by making separate but similar *personal* decisions to move in new directions—to seek more education, to aspire to higher positions in work outside the home, to structure their family lives in unprecedented ways. While a few women in previous cohorts (those already old) had made similar decisions, these women were forerunners; they were in the minority. Only with the current cohorts of young women did such decisions become pervasive. These cohorts have burst the floodgates of custom. Through these "floodgate cohorts" (another new concept, cf. Riley, 1982), new norms have been suddenly brought out into the open. They have become institutionalized. Sex role attitudes and behaviors are becoming transformed.

To be sure, substantial minorities of women still reject these changes, men seem to be lagging behind, and older working women today are still facing pervasive discrimination. Yet the trend toward sex equality is pressing upon social institutions to accommodate the new norms—through new family forms, changed work schedules that enable fathers to work inside as well as outside the home, job sharing, and the gradual blurring of the lines dividing education, work, and retirement. However far the changes go, many women are growing old in new roles and new social institutions. And we must ask: Will new family forms and falling birth rates leave older women of the *future* bereft of kin? Will those future older women who are still married (typically younger than their husbands) continue to work after their husbands retire, potentially creating a new family phase of "husband retirement"?

Changes in Sex Ratios

A second major change affecting women's lives is in sex ratios of successive cohorts (i.e., the number of men per 100 women). Among cohort members over age 65, the sex ratio was 102 in 1900; today it is under 70, that is, there are fewer than 70 males to every 100 females. Of course, one of the most drastic changes in human history is the century-long increase in longevity; and since this increase has been greater for women than for men, when we talk about contemporary older people, we are to a great extent talking about older women.

Thus in cohorts who are old today, there are striking differences between older men and women in their marital status and their living arrangements. Nearly eight out of ten elderly males are married and living with their spouses. By contrast, only just over one-third of females over age 65 are married and living with their husbands (Brody & Brock, in press). (For more details on demographic trends, see Somers, Chapter 2, infra.) How will older women of the *future* confront this last phase of life, the predictable phase of widowhood? Will many elderly widows live entirely alone, as they do today? Or will new forms of close relationships develop among women? New forms of congregate living? New norms accepting remarriage between older women and younger men following divorce or bereavement? Such questions demand the best efforts of social scientists.

Changes in Labor Force Participation

My third example of the effect of social change on the aging process—an example meriting our extended attention—concerns women's century-long movement away from complete domesticity and into the labor force. What can cohort analysis tell us about this transformation in the work life of women?

The most familiar data on female labor force participation are cross-sectional—that is, *not* analyzed by cohorts. Cross-sectional data correspond to the verticals in my imaginary diagram. They show, by age, the proportions of women in the labor force at particular periods. Such data are clearly important for many purposes (showing proportions of women actually working at various ages, the age-related match or mismatch between work roles available and women seeking work, the relations among workers of differing age, and so on). What these cross-sectional data do *not* describe are the work *lives* of women. Only when the data are rearranged by cohorts do they provide clues to the aging process. In my diagram, the cohort rearrangement corresponds to the diagonals. Let me tell you about seven successive cohorts of women, ranging from those born in about 1880 to those born about 1940, for which data are available (Riley, 1981a). For each cohort, a curve shows the life-course pattern of labor force participation.

Two aspects of these life-course curves are particularly interesting. First, for each more recent cohort, the entire curve is generally higher than its predecessor—reflecting the long-term rise in labor force participation. Second, these curves change shape from one cohort to the next. The earliest cohort (1880) starts with a peak at age 20 and then shows a gradual decline with aging. The middle cohorts (born around 1920 and 1930) show a peak at age 20, then a dip at age 30 (when the children are little) followed by a steep rise as women grow older. And the most recent cohorts (born around 1940) do not even show the dip around age 30 but tend to rise steadily from age 20 on. Thus there has been a complete reversal in the shape of these life-course curves—from a general *decrease* in participation over the life course of early cohort members, to a general *increase* in participation over the lives of more recent cohort members. Over the century, the work lives of women have been entirely altered.

When such data are observed, how can these striking cohort patterns be interpreted? Clearly, they have many important implications for women's lives, and they suggest a variety of questions for further study. Looking at any *single* cohort, we can ask why, on the average, *individual women* tend to work at certain ages (e.g., while young and unmarried) or not to work at other ages (e.g., when they have little children, or when they have grown old).

But when the several cohorts are compared, how can the striking *cohort differences* in life-course patterns be interpreted? Such changes across cohorts raise macro-level societal questions: How is it that many millions of women in one cohort have come to behave differently from many millions of women in another cohort? Why has the entire course of women's work life altered? Why have the age criteria for entering or leaving the work role shifted? Why are children no longer a major obstacle for today's women? In answering such questions, many broad social changes are potentially involved. For example, there has been a breakdown of *employers'* resistance against hiring older married women—as the number of female-typed jobs has expanded, and experience with older women has shown they can perform after all. Moreover, recent cohorts of women as *employees* have found it increasingly acceptable to work, learned to manage both work and family, come increasingly to seek added income—perhaps also to seek independence and self-fulfillment.

Not only the pattern but also the meaning of women's work has changed. Cohorts of women who worked at the beginning of the century were mainly the poorly educated, the young singles, the immigrants. Today, the higher a woman's educational attainment, the more likely she is to be in the labor force. And levels of educational attainment continue to rise.

What, then, do all these changes in women's working portend for the future? Save for current threats of unemployment, I have few doubts about the occupational future for those women choosing to work outside the home. Sizable proportions will increasingly play important roles as doctors, lawyers, scientists, technicians, business executives, nurses, politicians, diplomats, musicians, artists, and the like. As each new cohort passes through the changing social structure and grows into old age, women will have had more training, greater opportunity for lifetime earnings, and wider experience outside the household.

Changes in Cigarette Smoking

These three examples of cohort differences prompt me to consider one more that links directly to health. Cigarette smoking, the most deadly of the health risk factors, provides a dramatic and sobering example of how life-preserving behaviors can be responsive to policy changes in society. Over the past decades each successive cohort of adult *males* in the United States—presumably alerted by the Surgeon General's warnings—has been less likely than its predecessors to smoke (Riley, 1981a). For *women,* however—up until the health warnings of the mid-1960s—the proportions who smoked *increased* from cohort to cohort—in line with the "liberation" of women. Only after the widely broadcast Surgeon General's report did the most recent cohorts of women begin to follow the declining pattern of males. Thus predictably, the death rates attributable to smoking, currently increasing for women (Brody & Brock, in press) can be expected to decline as these more recent cohorts grow older.

Lessons from Cohort Analysis

These examples of massive cohort differences in life-course patterns raise heady questions which I cannot hope to deal with in this chapter. Yet I do believe that our cohort perspective gives us some handles on them. First, in looking ahead to the status of women in the shadowy future, we can at least hold to certain facts, since the characteristics and early experiences of women in cohorts already born are fully established. Second, cohort analysis underscores the wide variability and plasticity in the aging process—a fact that generates great hope for enhancing the lives of older women in the future. Third, going back to my imaginary diagram, the existence of numerous cohort differences alerts us to the dangers of ignoring them, to committing what I call the "life-course fallacy." Many studies commit this fallacy by simply comparing old people with young people at a given time (a vertical slice in the diagram), and then erroneously interpreting the cross-sectional *age differences* to refer to the process of aging over the life course. This fallacious reasoning has produced widespread, but false, stereotypes of inevitable aging decline.

For example, anyone who has read the geriatric literature is familiar with the classic diagrams (cf. Shock, 1977) which show a nearly linear decrease from age 30 to age 80 in such functions as nerve conduction velocity, heart output, and maximum breathing capacity. These findings are all too often interpreted as inevitable aging declines and accepted without question in medical textbooks. Yet they are based on cross-sectional studies, hence subject to a potential life-course fallacy. Who is to say that the cohorts of young women today, if they follow regimens of healthy living, will deteriorate in breathing capacity or heart output as rapidly in their old age as the cohorts who were old when this geriatric scrutiny began?

Meantime, without regard to the dangers of the cross-section fallacy, the stereotype of inevitable aging decline persists, extending to many presumed "age decrements" in sensation, perception, and ability to react quickly to stimuli. And the stereotype often becomes a self-fulfilling prophecy. For example, many physicians, because they look on aging as a process of inevitable and universal biological deterioration (Coe & Brehm, 1972), spend less time in office visits with older patients than with younger ones (Kane, Solomon, Beck, Keeler, & Kane, 1980), and give them less elaborate and drastic treatment (De Vita, 1980). Old people themselves also tend to accept this negative stereotype, to take their aches and pains for granted, and to seek palliative rather than preventive or corrective treatment (Kart, 1981; Riley & Foner, 1968). Such examples disclose the danger implicit in the persistently negative stereotypes of aging—the danger of giving up in the face of presumably inexorable deterioration, of not discovering how older people can live the later years of life to the full.

INTERVENTIONS

Let me conclude with some new research and some old exhortation. My parting question is this: What can be done right now about future cohorts? As we have seen, because society is continually changing, cohorts of women now young or middle-aged will almost certainly grow old in new ways. We must use these changes to ensure that their future lives are enhanced: partly through dispelling false stereotypes, but most importantly through deliberate interventions in social changes as they are taking place.

How, then, can this potential for optimization be realized? Clearly not exclusively through global imperatives to individuals simply to eat properly or to exercise regularly. Nor exclusively through individual modification of specific behaviors and attitudes toward immunization, avoidance of tobacco, moderate use of alcohol, or compliance with medical treatment when needed. Nor can the potential be fully met through societal provisions of safer highways or cleaner air and water. For research demonstrates that the quality of aging depends in large part also on the roles women perform in their ever-changing daily lives; on the nature of their family relations; on rewards or punishments from work and the ways women learn to cope with the combined pressures from job and household; on the support women receive from significant others and from health professionals, as losses of relatives and friends accumulate in old age; on women's attitudes toward death—both of self and of spouse. In short, the quality of aging depends on the subtle and continuing interplay between women growing older and the gradual accretion of fortunate or adverse circumstances in the day-to-day roles they perform in a changing society. And on the mechanisms of this continuing interplay through neural, sensorimotor, endocrine, immunological, and other physiological systems, all of which are themselves aging and can have direct impact on health and functioning.

Right now these concrete conditions and specific mechanisms of aging in women's daily lives are being affected by many social changes that can either enrich or diminish the quality of the later years. As strategic examples of these changes, two virtual revolutions are transforming both the process of aging and the environing social conditions: the revolution in longevity and the technological revolution that promises to permeate the workplace and the household with computers, robots, telecommunication, and information. Because both revolutions are going on around us, they are often overlooked. Yet as students of aging and social change, we are beginning to reckon with them, to harness them to our goal of optimizing the aging process for women, and hopefully also for men.

Implications of Longevity

Many early research findings are at hand to aid in this pursuit. Consider what we already know about longevity. The revolution in average length of life is unprecedented in all history. Over two-thirds of the world's improvement in longevity from prehistoric times until the present has taken place in the brief period since 1900 (Preston, 1976). In the United States, life expectancy at birth has risen from less than 50 in 1900 to well over 70 today— roughly 70 for men and 78 for women. And as most deaths now occur not in infancy and young adulthood but at the oldest ages (two-thirds of all deaths after age 65), life expectancy, contrary to earlier predictions, is continuing to increase most rapidly of all at age 85 and over (Brody & Brock, in press; Manton, 1982). The facts are familiar, but their full implications for the daily lives and functioning of older people are still elusive. Work life has been transformed; as people now spend at least one-quarter of their adult lives, not at work, but in retirement (Torrey, 1982: 184). Family life has been transformed, as people now live through a sequence of households, not only as child and then parent, but later also as grandparent and great-grandparent; as (apart from divorce) husbands and wives marrying at the customary ages can now expect to survive jointly for some 40 to 50 years; and as large numbers of people over 65 (most of them women) are caring for their own aged parents.

Lives have been extended, but role structures and opportunities for men as well as for women have been slow to catch up. At work, there are few new job opportunities for middle-aged and older women. In the household, most old people live alone (one-half of all women over age 75 live entirely alone—and while most elderly men are still married, most elderly women are widows; Brody et al., 1983). And because they have lost their traditional places in society, some old people feel useless, unappreciated, lonely—feelings that can lead to inactivity, apathy, or depression and thus contribute directly to physical and mental deterioration and disability.

It is this lag between increased longevity and role opportunity that has thwarted human development in the later years. It is in the provision of role opportunities for these extended lives that interventions and modifications are sorely needed. For given the opportunity for involvement and active pursuits, we know that most old people—men and women alike—maintain high levels of vigor and productivity; most cherish their independence and function effectively in the household. And we already know a good deal about particular interventions in social conditions, resources, and incentives that can sustain health and functioning even at the oldest ages.

Let me rehearse some of the research results in hand. For example, research shows that intellectual decline with aging (when it occurs) can often be slowed or reversed with opportunities for added practice, with instructions about strategies for approaching the problem, and with incentives that increase motivation and attention (Willis & Baltes, 1980). Several studies (Horn & Donaldson, 1980; Poon, Walsh-Sweeney, & Fozard, 1980) show that older people can often be taught to compensate for declines in reaction time, memory, and other age-related deficits (through mnemonic strategies, carefulness, and persistence); that physical training of older people can reduce anxiety and improve intelligence as well as physical well-being (Perlmutter, 1983); that illness can often be alleviated through social supports and improved coping behaviors (Cobb, 1979). We also have many clues that specific characteristics of the work role have striking consequences

for the aging process: that complexity of the job, lack of routini-
zation, or freedom from close supervision can, as people grow
older, enhance their intellectual functioning and their mental
(and ultimately their physical) well-being (Kahn, 1981; Kohn,
1981). And we know that many serious disabilities (even when
experienced in nursing homes) can be reduced by social regimens that reward activity and independence (Barton, Baltes, &
Orzech, 1980; Rodin, 1980). Thus the revolution in longevity
points to feasible and highly useful interventions.

The Implications of Technology

It is a new and exciting idea that the emerging technological
revolution may be providing the potential for introducing many
of these needed interventions. (As the Industrial Revolution extended the human body, the Technological Revolution is extending the human brain.) As this revolution is rapidly transforming
people's roles in both the workplace and the household, it will
most certainly affect the aging process—either positively or nega-
tively; and we in the National Institute on Aging are now hard
at work studying how the course of the revolution can be guided
positively toward our goal of extending health and effective functioning in the middle and later years. Already we have come upon
a provocative paradox here: the revolution in longevity is extending lives, but the technological revolution is sharply *curtailing* the
half-life of particular occupations and skills. This means that
periodic modification and relearning will be required of women
and men of all ages—not just of the old. In effect, the skills of
older women and older people generally will no longer be more
obsolete than those of younger people, since everyone will continually be starting afresh to catch up with the advancing technology and the proliferation of information.

 In a technological society, then, older women may be less
disadvantaged than at present. In addition, technology itself may
be variously useful in optimizing health and performance in later
life. As high technology is introduced into the workplace, we are
beginning to test hypotheses that possible negative consequences
can be avoided and that technological changes can, instead, be
designed constructively so as to challenge rather than inhibit workers, to allow independence rather than subordination, to vary
rather than routinize the tasks, and in some situations even to

reduce stress through telecommunicating rather than traveling from home to work. Similarly we are beginning to explore new uses for technology in the household that can help the frail elderly to function independently in such mundane matters as providing timepieces they can see, bathtubs they can use, jars they can open, stoves they can reach without burning themselves, signaling devices for help if needed (cf. Falletti, 1982). And on the high-technology front, robots are being developed to take over some of the difficult chores. Computer games are beginning to come on line for older people that can provide involvement, stimulation, and practice in rapid decision making. In such ways, I am proposing that technology can be made to operate positively as a stimulus to continuing vigor, and can be used as a prosthesis enabling the disabled to sustain their major activities.

I conclude this illustrative discussion of high technology to reemphasize the fundamental proposition with which I began: aging is not immutable but is rather subject to social intervention. This potential for technology as stimulus and prosthesis is just one instance of the challenge to all of us—in science, policy, or professional practice—to join forces in intervening in current social changes to optimize the daily lives of women (and men) who are growing older. We are gradually broadening the necessary knowledge base. Now we can make increasing use of what we already know about social change, aging, and health to postpone disability and dependency to the very last years of the extended life course.

This, I take it, is the objective of this book.

2
Toward a
Female Gerontocracy?
Current Social Trends

ANNE R. SOMERS

Three major trends are converging to produce a demographic revolution in the United States—the aging of the population, the growing proportion of women in the population, and the shrinking family.[1] Each of the three trends has been documented by the Bureau of the Census, the National Center for Health Statistics, and/or other demographers and social scientists. First, I will summarize the major facts and then go on to discuss some societal consequences, including the need for major adjustments in several areas.

THREE MAJOR TRENDS

Aging of the Population

Between 1900 and 1980 approximately 27 years were added to average life expectancy at birth, which is now over 73 years.

The median age of the population rose from 16 in 1800 and 23 in 1900 to 30 in 1980.

---

[1] The factual information in this paper is derived from various governmental sources, especially the Bureau of the Census, the National Center for Health Statistics, and the Social Security Administration. Where available, published data have been supplemented by more recent unpublished data. Useful compilations, especially relating to the elderly are contained in the following documents (see References): H. B. Brotman, *Every Ninth American*, 1982; C. Allan and Herman Brotman, *Chartbook on Aging in America*, 1981; and U.S. Department of Health, Education, and Welfare, 1975–79.

Even for the elderly, life expectancy has increased dramatically, especially in the last few decades. Between 1950 and 1980,
for example, about 2.5 years were added to the life expectancy
of the average 65-year-old American, more than were gained in the
50 years from 1900 to 1950.

In 1980, the average life expectancy for men of age 65 was
over 14 years; for women, nearly 19 years. By 2000, the average
woman of 65 can look forward to over 21 years.

The number of elderly in the population has increased from 3
million in 1900 to over 26 million in 1981, with Census Bureau
projections of 32 million in 2000 and 56 million in 2030. As percentages of total population, the rise has been from 4 in 1900 to
about 11.5 today, with projections to 20 percent or more as the
famous (some say infamous) World War II baby-boom cohort
reaches 65, starting about 2010.

Over one-fifth of all U.S. households were headed by persons
over 65 in 1980.

Not only is there an increase in the number and proportion of
those 65 and over, but of those 75+, and even 85+. The 75+ age-
group is the fastest growing in the nation. In 1900, there were less
than 1 million people in the United States over 75 years of age; in
1980 an estimated 9.5 million. As for those 85+, there were only
about 100,000 in 1900; 2.3 million in 1980; and a projected 4.6
million by 2010, a doubling of the present number. At that point,
these "old-old" individuals will constitute 13–15 percent of all
those over 65.

Growing Proportion of
Women in the Population

Historically, there were more men than women in the United
States, a situation that persisted through the early 1940s. Since
World War II, however, the reverse has been true. In 1981, the
population was 51 percent female.

Needless to say, the discrepancy is greater at the older ages.
For those 65 and over, the 1980 ratio was 148 women to 100
men; for those 85 and over, 224/100, expected to rise to 254/100
by 2000.

The improved life expectancy of black women and those of
other races has dramatically altered the traditional sex/race ratios.
The black woman of 65 has, today, an average life expectancy
four years longer than the average white man at that age.

The Shrinking Family

While marriage rates have changed very little during the twentieth century—fluctuating around 10 per 1000 population—the divorce rate has increased over sixfold—from 0.7 per 1000 to 5.3 per 1000. Over the past 20 years, the divorce ratio, that is, the number of divorced persons per 1000 persons who are married and living with a spouse, tripled. By 1981, the ratio for all women was 129 per 1000; for black women, 289 per 1000.

The size of the average household has declined significantly, from 3.14 persons in 1970 to 2.73 in 1981. In 1970, one-parent families accounted for 11 percent of all families with children; in 1981, 21 percent.

In 1981, 19 million individuals—23 percent of all households—lived alone. This was a 75 percent rise over 1970. The rise in "singles" has been greatest for the younger age-groups, that is, for those 25 to 34, about 300 percent. The latter figure presages the future.

Sixty-two percent of persons living alone in 1981 were women. Among these, the proportion divorced or never married rose while the proportion widowed declined.

Many additional demographic and economic trends could be cited. But the above is more than enough to substantiate my thesis: American society is gradually becoming not only a gerontocracy but a female gerontocracy, and increasingly a society of individuals living alone, with nonrelatives, or institutionalized, that is, without traditional family supports. The implications are enormous, not only for the individual, who faces a lengthy but increasingly dependent and probably lonely old age, but for society as a whole.

CLUES TO FUTURE
SOCIETAL CHANGES

What clues can we identify for future societal changes? Here are four areas in which distinctive needs and behavioral patterns, associated with age, sex, or both, may be identified: health and use of health services, income, the physical environment, and cultural and political values.

about 15 percent of their income on housing; those still paying a mortgage, over 25 percent; and renters nearly one-third. Nearly 16 percent of the rental units had serious physical inadequacies, according to the Department of Housing and Urban Development, compared to only 6 percent of units that were owned.

Data from the Law Enforcement Assistance Administration (LEAA) showed that some 2.2 million persons over 65 suffered crimes against their person or household in 1979. According to this source, the rate of victimization of the elderly is significantly less than for younger persons. For example, the personal victimization rate against women 65+ was 24 per 1000 compared to 125 per 1000 for women 14 to 64. For household crimes, the comparable rates were 103 per 1000 (both sexes) and 247 per 1000.

There is considerable evidence, however, that the crime problem may be substantially greater than indicated by the LEAA statistics. Older persons may be more fearful of reporting crimes than those who are younger. A number of local studies reveal higher rates, particularly among low-income, inner-city residents. The National Council on the Aging, Inc. (1976) revealed that one out of every four elderly persons fears crime as a very serious problem. Other studies substantiate this finding and point out the far-reaching consequences of this fear, affecting many aspects of daily life and health.

The trend for older women to live alone has clearly been a mixed blessing. The advantages are most obvious in the first years —the relief of not being a "burden" to one's children or younger siblings, the brief exhilaration of being a "free woman" again. But the "negatives" increase rapidly as the years go by—the high percentage of income that must go just for housing, especially in the case of renters, the gradually deteriorating physical conditions, the growing fear of crime and violence as one gets older and physically weaker, and the growing loneliness with all that implies for mental *and* physical health.

Cultural and Political Values

Religious affiliation and attendance at church or synagogue are higher among the elderly than any other age-group. A 1979 survey reported that almost all of those 65+ had at least a religious preference; only 3 percent did not. The elderly are a major resource for the churches of America, constituting nearly one-fourth of their membership, while the churches are an important source of community services and supports.

The formal educational level—as measured by years of schooling—of the average older American is rising but still surprisingly low. In 1952, only 18 percent had completed high school. By 1980, it was still only 38 percent. By 1990, it should reach one-half and perhaps one in ten will be college graduates.

Despite inadequacies of formal education, older Americans are surprisingly well informed. They are prime users of TV and newspapers, especially news and public affairs programs. After 65, 80 percent report daily viewing of TV news compared to only 48 percent of those 18 to 24. The elderly are the heaviest subscribers to daily newspapers.

Older persons are more likely to vote than younger ones. In the 1980 elections, for example, 65 percent of those 65+ voted, compared to 55 percent of those under 55 and 40 percent of those under 25. Although voting falls off after 75, 58 percent of this age-group voted in 1980. Older men had a better turnout than women—70 percent versus 61 percent.

The latter figure, however, obscures a very important new trend in American politics—the rapidly increasing preponderance of women in the voting electorate. Although there have been, for years, more women than men in every adult age bracket, this gender advantage was traditionally cancelled out by the men's better voting record. As late as 1964, the voting percentage of men was 72, of women 67. However, young women are now more likely to vote than young men and apparently they are carrying this pattern into the middle-age groups. By 1980, the historical distinction for the population as a whole had disappeared, with both sexes reporting about 59 percent. If this pattern persists as these younger women age, and given their tremendous numerical superiority in old age, the historical distinction will be significantly reversed and a "female gerontocracy" will indeed become operative—at least in the voting booth.

Will this change be reflected in substantive political issues? At least some informed commentators think it will. A recent article in the *New York Times*, based on Census Bureau Data, *Times*/CBS polls, interviews with the national chairmen of both major political parties and other responsible sources, concludes that "women, whose political attitudes used to be barely distinguishable from those of men, are beginning to take positions on issues that differ sharply from those taken by men. . . . Women have begun allying themselves more with Democratic positions" (Clymer, 1982, p. A1). These are changes, in the view of the *Times,* that "worry the Republicans and raise the long-range hopes of the Democrats."

The increasingly divergent views are most noticeable among young men and women. On the question of Social Security, for example, 49 percent of men of all ages said the Democrats would do a better job compared to 31 percent who preferred the Republican position. For men 18 to 24, the number had shifted to 46 and 35, respectively. By contrast, younger women favored the Democratic position on Social Security even more than all women. On national defense, all ages of men favored the Republican position while all ages of women favored the Democratic. Among younger persons, the same differences were even more pronounced.

To quote the *Times* (Clymer, 1982, p. D22), "From unemployment, to the military, to controlling federal spending to creating a 'budget that is fair to all the people,' women 18–44 were considerably more Democratic in their allegiances than were the men." Interestingly, these distinctions did not apply to such so-called women's issues as equal rights and abortion. On these two questions, the proportion of young men and young women who favored were just about the same; indeed, the men were slightly more in favor. Although the full implications of these trends remain to be seen, obviously, much more is at stake than simply women's rights.

Reviewing these various trends, the impact of the growing legions of elderly women on American society—already paradoxical—is difficult to predict for the future, and enormously intriguing. Most of the indices of individual well-being have improved substantially in recent years—at least up to 1980, after which we have few data. Nevertheless, the increase in the number and proportion of older women in the total population and their still relatively disadvantaged position with respect to many key indicators—health, jobs, income, formal education, family supports—suggests at least a temporary lowering of overall standards for the nation as a whole, particularly with respect to physical and material goods and values. At the same time, women's greater emphasis on religious and community values and activities, their greater interest in public affairs, and their better voting record suggest a greater commitment to ethical and humanistic values, as summarized in the Biblical injunction, "Love thy neighbor as thyself."

If the attitudes on major public issues and voting behavior of to-day's young women persist into old age, this latter trend could become highly significant.

However, before one leaps to the conclusion that, around 2010, America will emerge as a peace-loving Garden of Eden, with most of its citizens role-modeling themselves after Florence Nightingale or Mother Theresa, two important caveats are in order. First, the speed with which any of these changes will take place should not be exaggerated. The elderly today are only 11.5 percent of the population. In 2000 they will be only 12 percent. And women are still only 60 percent of this 11–12 percent. The U.S. is still far from "a female gerontocracy."

Second, and perhaps even more important, we can never forget that the production of wealth has to precede the sharing of wealth. It was Gunnar Myrdal, one of the foremost spokesmen for the Swedish welfare state, who said that affluence is a prerequisite to the welfare state. In our concern for dependency and assurance of security, we cannot afford to forget the importance of individual initiative, risk-taking, capital formation, and plain hard work. Nor should we ever conclude that the federal government is the only effective instrument for assuring security or that any one political party has a monopoly on wisdom or compassion. Any effort on the part of the elderly to claim an unreasonable proportion of the national income for too many years must, and will, be resisted by those who are younger and more productive of material wealth. What will be desparately needed, in this as in so many other areas, is a balance between the values and the talents of maturity and those of youth, of men and of women, of individual initiative and of collective or social security.

AREAS OF NEEDED ADJUSTMENT

This is neither the time nor the place to attempt any in-depth discussion of the many adjustments that will have to be made in American society if this creative balance is to be achieved, and if the profound trends noted in this chapter are to be assimilated or accommodated in a relatively peaceful and painless manner. I conclude by suggesting six adjustments that appear to me among the most urgent, elaborating only on the first.

1. *Redefinition of "old age."* Our conventional definition, accepted uncritically by almost everyone, places the dividing line at 65 and assumes that everyone over 65 is "aged." If this was true in Bismarck's day, when life expectancy was about 43, then it is patent nonsense today, when the average woman of 65 has a life expectancy of nearly 19 years, the average man over 14 years. If we expect society to provide us with adequate pensions, housing, health services, and other "old age" benefits, we will have to accept a more realistic definition of "old age."

    As one who believes that older people can, and should be encouraged to work as long as possible, for reasons of health as well as economics, and that compulsory retirement should be eliminated insofar as possible, I also believe that the normal pension age should be raised, both in terms of Social Security and private pensions. Provision for the sick or disabled, and for those who work in exceptionally dangerous or exhausting jobs, should be made through disability and early retirement programs. But the basic definition of "old age" should be gradually raised, in accordance with increasing life expectancy, certainly to at least 68 within a generation. Needless to say, for this policy to be effectively implemented, we will need something approaching full employment.

2. *Strengthening the Social Security system* for the future by protecting it both from irresponsible cutbacks or other political manipulation and from irresponsible demands by current beneficiaries.

3. *Development of various forms of congregate or shared housing* to meet the physical, security, and emotional needs of the elderly, especially the growing legions of elderly "singles," and at the same time help to revitalize many urban and rural ghettos, and provide a new market for the housing industry.

4. *Strengthen Medicare* for the future by adding preventive and long-term care services and introducing reasonable but effective cost controls.

5. *Strengthen state and local governments and clarify the appropriate federal role* through a thorough review of existing federal/state/local responsibilities and resources,

especially with respect to Medicaid and other health, housing, and welfare programs.
6. *Strengthen and stabilize the U.S. role in world affairs* by
   clearer definition of our foreign policies, economic as well
   as political, and by more restrained and more cost-effective
   use of military resources.

3
The Natural Superiority
of Women

IRVEN DEVORE AND
C. OWEN LOVEJOY

Are women naturally superior to men? The question is certainly one that will produce an instant response in a large segment of the general population. Some women would reply emphatically "yes," and some would reply with equal certainty "no." Interestingly, there are probably more men who would fall into the latter category than the former, if asked the same question. There would also certainly be a large segment of respondents who would immediately object to the *question,* and would reply to the effect that neither sex can be regarded as superior. As the title of this chapter implies, we are not among those who regard the question as unanswerable.

A fundamental question of this type requires some discussion of the methods that will be used to obtain its answer. In biology, there are essentially two methods by which one can resolve a major issue. First, one can argue from available data, weigh each point, and arrive at a conclusion. A second method, and one that is heuristically superior, is to rely on fundamental biological principles and arrive at an answer by induction.

More often than not, attempts to answer important biological questions fall into the first of the above two categories. One is familiar with long lists of attributes believed to be, by their prognosis, evidence in favor of the superiority of one sex or the other. Males are stronger and larger. Opponents to the male position then respond that while males can produce greater levels of musculoskeletal *force,* females are in many ways more resilient to major forms of catastrophic illness (e.g., atherosclerosis, heart disease, etc.), have greater longevity, and are therefore actually "stronger" than men. Such proposals and counterproposals are most likely to proceed without resolution. There are, of course, certain basic biological facts that *do* seem to be more definitive than others. Genetic defects that are sex-linked recessives (color blindness, Christmas disease, etc.), for example, will occur in females only at a rate equal to the square root of their male frequency; in this case females are clearly superior, and their advantage is directly linked to the genetic basis of sex determination. But there might be male counterarguments. The discussion could prove endless.

The second method of resolution, therefore, must be recruited. In addition to being a more decisive approach, it is also far more interesting than the more restrictive, evidentiary approach. In modern times, the most fundamental goal of science—explanation—all too frequently has been cast aside in favor of purely statistical argument. Frequently, we find ourselves bound to an unproductive "scientific method" simply because it is the "correct" procedure. Those presenting vast amounts of data coupled with sophisticated analytical methods are often more likely to convince their audience than those who provide an inductive argument from basic biological principle. In the final analysis, however, even more data may be collected, and the original conclusions overturned. To the contrary, if an argument from a fundamental and immutable biological principle is extended by cautious, logical procedure, the conclusions generated are equally as immutable as the underlying principle. No amount of data collection and compilation of fact could possibly answer a question so fundamental as the natural superiority of women. This question *must* be addressed by reference to the most basic tenets and axioms of biology, and we will therefore use this approach.

SEX

If we are to determine the superiority of one sex over another, then we are naturally first required to investigate the nature of the category itself. Why is there sex?

The smallest organisms on this planet reproduce *asexually*. By simple cell division, which can take place rapidly in such organisms, a single cell may produce millions of offspring, identical to itself, in a relatively short time span. Natural selection, which is the most fundamental axiom of modern biology, is synonymous with *reproductive success*: the organism that reproduces most effectively leaves the greatest number of descendants. Since biological space is always limited, those descendants will eventually be the only contributors to succeeding generations. This is the nature of selection and the evolutionary process.

Since reproductive success is the arbiter of extinction versus survival, an obvious corollary is that every individual organism will invest as much energy as possible in the process of reproduction. In sexual reproduction, however, offspring carry only one-half of their mother's genotype. Why do females genetically share their offspring with males? The uninitiated might regard the question as supercilious: "They must share—males are required for reproduction." To the contrary, as pointed out above, many organisms are genderless.

A variety of beetles, moths, sow bugs, flies, shrimp, salamanders, and fish are capable of *parthenogenesis*: direct female replication with no male genetic contribution. The Amazon molly (*Mollienesia formosa*), so frequently an inhabitant of the amateur's fish tank, is a prime example. All mollies are females. They attract males of closely related species, which inseminate them. The eggs of these fish require spermatozoa for stimulation, but the nuclei of the sperm are then ejected, and the resulting progeny are all genetically identical to their mother. Kallman (1962) studied a colony of these fish and found that close to 80 percent were descendent from only two individuals!

If males are not required for reproduction, why do they exist? The molly is a perfect example with which to answer this question. Environments are constantly changing. In fact, as we too often forget, the most important environmental constitutents are other organisms. We can deal easily with rain, cold, wind, and humidity, but far less well with bacteria, viruses, and predators. Our foodstuffs are all organisms. Since natural selection is constantly acting on all these elements of our environment, the result is a writhing cauldron of evolutionary activity. Adaptive vigilance is requisite, and new adaptations require genetic and phenotypic variation. Eighty percent of the mollies in the above colony were of only two genotypes, so there was virtually no genetic variation from which to select, if environmental change were to demand it.

Other organisms provide illustrative examples of how parthenogenesis can be advantageously mixed with sexual reproduction. The common aphid is an excellent choice (well known to any reader who has ever attempted a rose garden). A single female can produce more than 500 billion offspring. She achieves this by parthenogenesis. In fact, during the time her daughter offspring is developing within her, there is another generation developing within the daughter! Within a week's time a single aphid can reproduce millions of offspring (and if one doesn't spot the infestation, he/she[1] may very well wave goodbye to the "General Lee's" or whatever other rose varieties in the garden). The drawback to this process is that all of the aphid offspring are genetically identical. If the insecticide you've chosen is effective, it will be equally effective against every offspring—there is no genetic variety from which to select resistance. But aphids have solved this problem as well. As winter approaches, they begin to produce both male and female offspring. The offspring of different parents sexually reproduce, and genetic variation is instilled for presentation to the novel environmental demands of the next summer season (your new brand of insecticide).

At this point we can pause to consider some implications of the above discussion. If there is only one gender capable of physical replication, that gender is primary. Thus the female gender is fundamental and the male auxiliary. Males were "invented" by natural selection as a means of providing genetic variety. Moreover, whenever the environment allows it, that is, is relatively stable (as in the case of the Amazon molly), or is seasonally stable (as in the case of aphids), and temporarily ceases to require genotypic variety, females of many species can regress to asexual reproduction.

That evolutionary success is axiomatic and females are the primary gender is one obvious corollary. Another is as follows: a female is most successful if she can produce more offspring than any other female of her species. Returning to the aphids described above, it is clear that this requirement can often be met without male contribution. By means of parthenogenesis, she can reproduce an enormous number of offspring, each identical to herself, but if a single genetic deficiency is present, all will be reproductively inferior to the offspring of other females. So she makes a sacrifice: she mates with a male. When this occurs (because of the chromosomal grouping of genes and the process of crossover), each fertilized ovum she produces becomes an adult organism genetically distinct from all others. She has invested only

---

[1] The order in which personal pronouns are presented is troublesome; here we list them alphabetically.

half her genetic identity in her offspring, but she has invested that "half-identity" in a vast pool of genetic variety. The almost universal role of sexual reproduction among higher organisms demonstrates that this strategy is better than investing in simple self-replication.

One might therefore conclude that a strict reliance on the process of sexual reproduction (as in mammals, for example) elevates the male to a state of equality with the female gender. Such, however, is not the case. Females remain the only gender capable of replication and although males are now required for that process, because only the female carries out embryogenesis, that role can be quite transitory. In addition, only one male is required for fertilization of many females. This creates a surplus of males, that is, the male *gender* is required, but only a few of its representatives are needed—males are reproductively inexpensive and as such are easily manipulated by selection. In fact, selection tends to accelerate the reduction of reproductive value in the single male.

The basic male strategy is the same as that of the female—produce as many offspring as possible. This favors fertilization of as many females as possible, and the greater the number of females that can be successfully fertilized by a single male, the more prevalent his offspring (and their behavior) become. The result is even more surplus males, and an even lower reproductive value of each individual male.

Any female who makes the genetic sacrifice of sexual reproduction can recoup some of her genetic loss by actively "choosing" a male (from the large pool available) with whom to mate. A female will produce both male and female offspring, and *both* genders will carry half her genetic identity. Her future reproductive success will be directly correlated to that of her male offspring (in spreading her genes in future gene pools). What kind of male offspring should she create? The answer is obvious—she must produce males with the greatest reproductive potential—the greatest chance at success in fertilizing females in the next generation. Obviously a female cannot directly reshuffle her genetic material toward achieving this goal. She can, however, do the next best thing—*choose* a male who most closely meets the "desired" reproductive profile. Thus an important corollary of sexual reproduction is the primary role of female choice: females must actively select those males with the greatest reproductive potential.

HIGHER ORGANISMS:
MAMMALS AND BIRDS

The most complex and highly evolved organisms on our planet are mammals and birds. They live exclusively by consumption of other organisms and tend to reside near the apex of the food pyramid. They have relatively large brains, and rely on learning and complex (including social) behavior for survival. They are the product of tens of millions of years of *anagenesis,* which is the process by which an organism evolves increasingly greater control of its own environment—it becomes more and more reliant on homeostasis, and less dependent on environmental perturbations. Thus both mammals and birds control their body temperature, live in social groups of conspecifics, locate food with complex sensory mechanisms, etc. Mammals, in addition, carry their embryos internally and provide special postnatal food for optimum growth.

Despite their complexity, however, the fundamental rules of sexual reproduction are still completely applicable. The female still achieves reproductive success by leaving more offspring than other females of the same species, and therefore by choosing males most likely to provide her descendents with the highest reproductive potential. Generally, *male* strategy varies along a continuum with two distinct poles. At one end of this continuum is intense formalized competition with other males [often during a proscribed breeding season determined, of course, by females *(tournament sex)*]; at the other is permanent social bonding with a single female *(pair bonding)* coupled with intensive parental care by both sexes. Most mammals fall near the former pole and most birds fall near the latter.

Where a mammalian or bird species falls on this continuum is, of course, determined by the female. As just pointed out, these higher organisms are complex and homeostatic. They require relatively long periods of subadult development and their heavy reliance on learning and social behavior require relatively intense parenting and a long subadult learning period. These features require female strategy to be a compromise between the quantitative and qualitative strategies of reproduction. The continuum described above is simply the result of the degree to which one or the other of these two methods is dominant in overall species strategy.

While bird strategy usually falls at one end of the continuum, this is not always the case, and they thus provide us with instructive examples of each strategy. The albatross provides an excellent illustration of the qualitative pole. They are very large birds and have ranges of thousands of miles, and this allows them to nest in places of maximum safety. The young are altricial and require constant feeding and care. So much energy is required in their production that the female can afford to bear only one young at a time and more than a full year of postnatal care is required before her offspring is independent. Whether or not she is reproductively successful depends on the quality of care her single offspring is provided during its development. What kind of male will she choose? If she chooses one that tends toward polygynous, competitive behavior, she retains the advantage of male offspring with the tendency to "spread" her genes in future generations, but only if they survive. To the contrary, if she chooses a male that will faithfully provision and care for her fledgling, she loses the advantage of promiscuity in her male offspring but she gains the advantage of *doubling* each of her infant's chances of survival. Which strategy is more effective depends on a variety of factors, too numerous to discuss here. One, however, is of particular importance—survivorship. How good an investment is each offspring? Albatrosses have life spans of over 60 years, and few predators. A female can thus have tremendous success if she steadily produces strong, healthy, well-socialized offspring (both male and female) that are active breeders. Albatross females choose males who mate for life, are active providers, and who are least likely to abandon them. She must be assured of these characters in the male she chooses, however, and as a consequence females have fostered elaborate courtship rituals. In birds that pairbond for life (such as the albatross), complex courtship behavior has evolved to "cement" the pairbond. Lorenz once commented that the gray lag goose becomes lovesick when her/his mate is absent. Loss of mate evokes depression, while reunion after a long separation elicits virtual ecstasy.

There are tournament strategists among birds as well. Domestic fowl (or more properly their undomesticated antecedent species) are a good example. Their young are precocial and develop rapidly, requiring relatively minimal care. The female therefore opts for a numerically superior strategy. Why? Once more, a complete answer would require a too lengthy discussion, but one obvious factor is their economic strategy. They rely heavily on seeds and worms plucked from the ground surface and their body size requires a considerable intake. Their ranges are small and they are poor flyers. They are thus constantly subject to predation, and even if they had the genetic potential to be long-lived (which they don't), their chances of reaching "old-age" are relatively small. A single offspring is therefore a poor reproductive investment. These factors have led the females to select highly competitive males who take little interest in their offspring. By selecting the numeric strategy their best opportunity for reproductive success is via male offspring that will dominate other males and inseminate a large number of females.

While most mammals are relative quantitative strategists, many are not. The North American beaver is a good example of a pair-bonding mammal. Again, some of the essential determinants of the chosen strategy are clear. They are slow-developing, long-lived, highly social rodents. These factors have led females to adopt the pair-bonding strategy and consequently to select males with the "appropriate" mating and parenting behavioral profile.

HOMO SAPIENS

But what of women—which is the topic at hand. Do females of our species conform to the above axioms and corollaries? What mating strategy have they selected? Obviously culture and other forms of nongenetic behavior are intensely critical in determining how females (and males) of our species behave, including their choice of mating strategy. Both of us believe, however, that there are still significant genetic undercurrents in modern human behavior, and that an understanding of such factors as the mating strategy of our immediate forebears is both instructive and illuminating. Only one of us, however, is of the opinion that the evidence for pair-bonding in early and modern man[2] is unusually strong. For obvious reasons[3], we will pause to briefly consider some of that evidence.

---

[2] The use of the generic term "man" will probably *engender* considerable criticism. However, it follows a long period of historical development in which it has attained a status of complete equivalency with *Homo sapiens*, i.e., it is the common name for our species. We thus use it without sexual connotation.

[3] The junior author, who is the one who believes this, is writing this part of the chapter.

We are, of course, primates. More specifically, we are higher primates. Higher primates are highly intelligent, very long-lived, slowly maturing mammals with extremely altricial infants. One would almost immediately conclude from this list of attributes that primates must be pair-bonding, qualitative strategists. But they aren't. Most primate species are polygynous and have substantially unequal sex ratios. Again the reasons for this apparent paradox are multiple and complex, but a primary one is the intense social behavior of primates. Most primates live in multimale groups with a strong dominance hierarchy, but one coupled with a less than complete reproductive isolation of females by any single male. Male behavior in primate troops is a complex combination of both tournament and parental-investment strategies. When, as rarely happens among higher primates, group behavior is *not* the norm, one end or other of the continuum tends to emerge. Thus the solitary orangutan is in many ways a tournament strategist, whereas the nuclear family-dwelling gibbon displays classic pair-bonding. But what is the primary strategy of man?

Our closest living relatives are chimpanzees, whose sexual strategy is often categorized as promiscuity, but which is exceedingly complex. Chimpanzees display some polygynous-like behaviors as well as some monogamous-like behaviors. It is sufficient here to simply state that the role of the supra-familial social group is so paramount that these various elements are combined into a unique sexual strategy that conforms to general principle, but not to easy categorization. Humans, however, are even more specialized than chimpanzees. We are more long-lived (few mammals and no other primates live as long as we), have the most altricial infants of any organism, have larger brains, and rely more intensely on learning than any other mammal. All of these things favor a pair-bonding strategy, yet a definitive answer remains elusive. Most pre-urban "anthropological" populations practice polygyny. At the same time, however, man is anatomically adorned with many of the classic parasexual attributes of a pair-bonding species (Lovejoy, 1981). We cannot attempt an answer here because we must quickly return to the immediate question at hand. Suffice it to say, however, that there is strong evidence for pair-bonding in early (and recent) man, but that this evidence must be viewed from the background of extreme social complexity, which tends to favor a mixture of characters from the qualitative-quantitative continuum.

THE NATURAL SUPERIORITY
OF WOMEN

By now the reader may be wondering just when we will turn to the question of the superiority of women. If this is the case, our earlier discussions have failed, because we have set forth incontrovertable evidence in favor of such a conclusion. Women are female mammals. As such, not only they, but an unbroken chain of generations preceding them, have been inescapably subject to the rules of evolution as set forth in its fundamental axioms and corollaries. The female gender is primary in *Homo sapiens* just as it is in all other species.

Does this make women naturally superior? Yes. Take any biological question and apply the axioms and corollaries defined above, and you will always arrive at this conclusion. Take for example, longevity. Who lives longer: men or women? The reader might be tempted to abandon this chapter and turn to an actuarial table for an answer. As pointed out in our beginning paragraphs, however, this will provide no satisfaction. In some cultures women will live longer, in others men. In most cases cultural variables (stress, taboos, eating habits, exposure to pathogens, etc.) will be found to heavily influence the available data to such an extent that a satisfactory answer cannot be reached with confidence as to which sex is actually *capable* of greater longevity.

We can, however, apply the principles outlined above. The longer a woman lives, the more children she can produce. Selection constantly favors increased longevity in women. The reader will object that women experience menopause and continue to survive beyond reproductive age. Apply your principles. This simply tells us that, for the greater part of that time our species has existed, so few women have survived to this age, that selection has been powerless to extend the length of the reproductive period.

Again, the reader might object, pointing out that the longer a male lives the more offspring *he* will leave. This is, of course, true, and will certainly be a selective factor in male longevity. However, the key factor is the total number of offspring. In fact, a male who fathers ten offspring early in life has a greater fitness than one who fathers ten in his lifetime. His offspring (as well as *their* offspring) will progressively replace those of older breeders in subsequent generations (all other factors being equal). Thus males tend to mature more quickly than females. So what will be the course of selection? It will follow the most effective course at the cost of the less effective. A male who fathers a large number of children early in his life will have a high fitness, even if he fails to achieve longevity. On the other hand, the female's reproductive rate is linear with age, and she must survive in order to achieve her full reproductive potential. Why are androgens responsible for early maturation and increased musculoskeletal development, but implicated in reduced longevity? The answer should be clear.

No matter what topic we might pick for application of our principles, the answer will always remain the same. Women are always more reproductively valuable than men, will always constitute the primary gender, and will always direct (via natural selection) the adoption of mating and reproductive strategies. The axioms and corollaries of evolution will always apply, whether we consider longevity, or resistance to disease or stress, or whatever.

Before concluding, however, two additional points seem worthy of mention. First, we must emphasize that gender is only one physical character and is the product of a single chromosome. A vast number of characters are autosomal and are thus equivalent in both sexes.

Last, a comment on the effects of pair-bonding and male parenting. In those species in which pair-bonding is established as the norm, it is instructive to note the benefits to the male gender. It is the *one* mating strategy in which the male is virtually elevated to a reproductive value equivalent to that of the female. In such species the sex ratio approximates unity and males become indispensable for successful reproduction. Under these conditions selection will be as favorable to the male as the female gender, and most of the above principles will apply equally to both sexes. Thus we conclude that while males can never be naturally superior to women, they can approach equality. It is most instructive that realization of equality requires intensification of male parenting behavior. Perhaps it is time that a *valid* form of "social Darwinism" be given consideration in modern sociological theory.

PART II
PHYSICAL HEALTH ISSUES

Many physical health issues are similar for older women and older men. These, while important, are not the focus of this book. In the following section, Verbrugge first points up gender differences from the epidemiological perspective, using mortality rates and statistics regarding chronic conditions and long-term disabilities. While women are far more durable than men in terms of number of years of survival, Verbrugge provides disquieting information about the quality of women's longer life span. Older women are about twice as likely as men to have arthritis, and 13 percent of elderly women experience limitations in their daily activities due to their arthritis. Each year, one in five aged women suffer an injury requiring medical attention, and their injury rate surpasses that of aged men—a reversal of the situation for younger men and younger women. The physical health picture painted by Verbrugge's epidemiological approach depicts older women as more often ill and experiencing more days of bed-disability, yet living longer than older men.

Lindsay's chapter then moves to one body system, the skeletal, to elucidate causes of some of the injuries to which Verbrugge referred. Bone loss, osteoporosis, in postclimacteric women is shown as a cause of the disproportionate number of painful and disabling fractures of the vertebral bodies, the neck of the femur, and of the wrist, experienced by older women. Indeed, almost 25 percent of women who reach the age of 80 will have experienced a fracture attributable to osteoporosis. Lindsay describes state-of-the-art methods for measuring bone mass and reports some promising research about preventing the occurrence of bone loss. Calcium supplementation, exercise, and certain hormonal therapies have been studied and found to contribute to the maintenance of bone mass.

39

In the final chapter in this section, Greenblatt and colleagues strike a hopeful note advocating long-term treatment of bone loss as well as other postclimacteric disorders with natural estrogens. They review the entire endocrine system, and the functions of the various endocrine glands in aged women, pointing out that the ovary is the only one to show regression in normal aging.

This section on physical health issues fittingly closes with Greenblatt et al.'s proposal to consider ovarian regression with its attendant bone loss, sexual dysfunction, and other uncomfortable correlates, as a treatable condition. Thus helping older women "grow old with grace and dignity" becomes a viable objective in their physical health care.

M. S.

4
An Epidemiological Profile of Older Women

LOIS M. VERBRUGGE

The United States population is becoming demographically old, and among the elderly more feminine. The rising number and percentage of older women has prodded scientists to study their problems and satisfactions, and policymakers to consider how the well-being of contemporary and future women aged 65+ can be enhanced.

This chapter discusses the physical health status of contemporary older women. We begin with longevity and mortality, reviewing the life expectancy of women who reach older ages and recent trends in their mortality rates. This tells us about the amount of life older women can expect, and their risks of its termination. Next, to get a better view of the quality of life, we look extensively at data on physical health, especially chronic conditions and long-term disability due to poor health. We do not discuss mental or nutritional health. These three aspects of health (physical, mental, nutritional) are certainly entwined, probably more closely for elderly persons than younger ones, but the goal here is to offer a comprehensive view of one aspect. Then, comparing the mortality and physical health data, we find that older women often have worse health status than older men, yet they live longer. This seems contradictory, but the explanation is actually a simple one. Finally, we speculate about the health of older women in the future. Compared to contemporary women, how will future cohorts feel on a daily basis? Can they anticipate less disability before death and longer lives?

The analysis is enhanced if we compare older women with other age-sex groups. Differences between older women's and older men's health reflect risks from their different roles and health habits throughout life, and also biological vulnerabilities related to sex. Differences between older women's and middle-aged women's health can reflect typical changes as people age, but also different life experiences and habits that cohorts have had (see Chapter 1). In this chapter, we choose to emphasize sex differences and will suggest aspects of older men's and women's lives that have led to different health outcomes for them.

Data are drawn mainly from national vital statistics and national health surveys. The mortality data encompass the entire population of people 65+, whether they are in institutions or not at time of death. The health data refer to noninstitutionalized people. About 5 percent of older people reside in institutions, often because of health problems. If they were included in health surveys, prevalence and disability rates would increase. (For data on health status of nursing home residents, most of whom are elderly, see Hing, 1981.)

MORTALITY OF OLDER WOMEN

Women who reach age 65 can expect to live about 18 more years (Table 4.1). This is true for both white and all other races. If they reach age 75, women can anticipate 12 more years of life.[1] Older men's life expectancy is lower at all ages; they have an average of 14 more years at age 65, and 9 years at age 75. Even at age 85, men's life expectancy is 1½ years less than comparable women's. These differences are direct outcomes of men's higher mortality rates at older ages; their rates are higher than women's at all ages under 65 as well. Thus, out of 100,000 males who are born, a smaller percent ever reach age 65 (69% vs. 83% for females, using current mortality rates), and their risks of death after 65 continue to be higher. Currently, men 65 to 69 die at twice

---

[1] Note that at these very elderly ages, all other women have higher life expectancy than white women do. This unusual "crossover" effect may be due to age inflation on death certificates for all Other women, or to a special hardiness of all other women who reach that age. Research suggests that the second reason is the main one (Manton, Poss, & Wing, 1979; Nam, Weatherby, & Ockay, 1978; Vaupel, Manton, & Stallard, 1979).

Table 4.1
Mortality of Older Women and Older Men,
by Race, United States 1978

	Life Expectancy[a]				
	e_{65}	e_{70}	e_{75}	e_{80}	e_{85}
All Races					
Females	18.4	14.7	11.5	8.9	6.9
Males	14.0	11.1	8.7	6.9	5.5
Sex difference (F–M)	4.4	3.6	2.8	2.0	1.4
Whites					
White females	18.4	14.8	11.5	8.8	6.7
White males	14.0	11.1	8.6	6.7	5.3
Difference	4.4	3.7	2.9	2.1	1.4
All others					
All other females	18.0	14.8	12.5	11.5	9.9
All other males	14.1	11.6	9.8	8.8	7.8
Difference	3.9	3.2	2.7	2.7	2.1

		Mortality Rates for All Causes				
		(Deaths per 100,000 population per past year)				
	Ages	65–69	70–74	75–79	80–84	85+
All races						
Females		1,685	2,725	4,713	7,509	13,541
Males		3,439	5,242	8,066	11,597	17,259
Sex ratio (M/F)		2.04	1.92	1.71	1.54	1.27
Whites						
White females		1,628	2,612	4,564	7,607	14,079
White males		3,394	5,167	7,996	11,822	18,100
Ratio		2.08	1.98	1.75	1.55	1.29
All others						
All other females		2,150	3,980	6,621	6,373	8,449
All other males		3,815	5,984	8,724	9,420	10,678
Ratio		1.77	1.50	1.32	1.48	1.26

Source: National Center for Health Statistics (1980a). Advance Report, Final Mortality Statistics, 1978. *Monthly Vital Statistics Report, Vol. 29,* No. 6 (Supplement 2), 17 September.
[a]Life expectancy (e_x) is the average remaining years of life for a person age x.

the rate women those ages do. Men's excess risk diminishes in their 70s and 80s; for the age-group 85+, men's rates are only 27 percent higher than women's.

As people enter their 70s and 80s, death rates rise steeply. They actually rise more sharply for women. It is as if women "catch up" as they approach the limits of human life.[2] Although women's risk of dying at every age remains less than men's, the pace quickens more rapidly from year to year. The subjective impact must be quite striking; elderly women see their female friends dying rapidly after age 70, and they probably become keenly aware of their own accelerating risks.

Trends since 1940 show that mortality rates have dropped more for older women than for older men (Fingerhut, 1982). From 1940 to 1978, the death rate for women 65+ declined by almost half (46.7%, age-adjusted). The gains occurred at all older ages (65–69, 70–74, etc.) and mainly in two time periods (1940–1954 and 1968–present). For older men, rates dropped 24.5 percent from 1940 to 1978. Similar to women, their gains occurred in all age-groups and were concentrated in the same two periods. Because of these declines, life expectancy for older people has risen since 1940: Women age 65 can expect 4.8 years more than their peers in 1940, and women age 75, 3.5 years more. The gain is smaller for men: 1.9 years for those age 65, and 1.5 for those age 75. (For the 1940 figures, see Grove and Hetzel, 1968: Table 50.)

After decades of continuous decline in U.S. mortality rates, rates stabilized in the 1950s. In the late 1960s, mortality rates began to drop again, and there is no sign that they will stop soon. From 1968 to 1978, death rates for females (All Ages) dropped 20 percent, and for males, 17 percent. Older people have benefited greatly in this recent period: For women, rates fell 20 percent (ages 65–74), 16 percent (75–84), and 27 percent (85+); for men, 17 percent, eight percent, and 21 percent for the same age-groups. Absolute changes in the rates are amazing; for example, mortality rates for women aged 65 to 74 dropped from 2681 per 100,000 to 2138. That means about 500 more women per 100,000 in those ages survive each year. Table 4.2 shows mortality rates in 1968 and 1978 for age-sex groups of older people.

[2] The maximum possible age to which a human can live is probably about 110 years (Fries & Crapo, 1981). This is called the human life span, and it will probably not change much even if mortality rates fall. More people will simply die near this limiting age than before. A different notion is maximum life expectancy. This is the average age at death in a society with lowest possible death rates. It is probably about 85. The current U.S. mortality projections assume that mortality rates will continue to drop but not reach "lowest possible" levels. By the year 2050, U.S. females may have a life expectancy at birth of 81 years; and men 72 years (U.S. Department of Commerce, 1977a).

Table 4.2
Mortality Rates for Older Women and Older Men, from All Causes and the Three Leading Causes, United States 1968 and 1978

| | Deaths per 100,000 population per year | | | | | | Percent Change (1968–1978) | | |
| | 1968 | | | 1978 | | | | | |
Ages	65–74	75–84	85+	65–74	75–84	85+	65–74	75–84	85+
All causes									
Females	2,681	6,978	18,425	2,138	5,863	13,541	−20%	−16%	−27%
Males	5,049	10,215	21,732	4,185	9,385	17,259	−17	− 8	−21
Diseases of heart									
Females	1,141	3,259	8,850	823	2,666	6,674	−28	−18	−25
Males	2,258	4,653	10,078	1,762	4,064	7,991	−22	−13	−21
Malignant neoplasms (Cancer)									
Females	553	869	1,224	589	959	1,139	+ 7	+10	− 7
Males	998	1,520	1,936	1,077	1,849	2,137	+ 8	+22	+10
Cancer of lung									
Females	39	50	55	85	87	70	+118	+74	+27
Males	306	293	194	389	479	317	+27	+63	+63
Cerebrovascular Diseases (stroke)									
Females	352	1,249	3,618	208	866	2,298	−41	−31	−36
Males	483	1,418	3,592	290	984	2,244	−40	−31	−38

Source: Fingerhut, L. A. Changes in Mortality Among the Elderly: United States, 1940–78. *Vital and Health Statistics*. Series 3, No. 22. Hyattsville, Md.: National Center for Health Statistics, 1982.

These recent gains appear for all but one of the leading causes of death for older people: diseases of heart, cerebrovascular diseases, influenza/pneumonia, arteriosclerosis, diabetes, accidents, bronchitis/emphysema/asthma, cirrhosis of the liver, and nephritis/nephrosis. Malignant neoplasms are the exception: After a period of stable rates, cancer mortality is now rising for older women, due especially to rises in lung cancer. Older men's cancer rates have been rising for decades; the recent period continues that trend with especially large increases in colon cancer. Lung cancer rates also climbed for men, but less rapidly than in prior decades and less rapidly than women's. In sum, the pace of rising cancer mortality has slowed for older men but has accelerated for older women. (Table 4.2 shows the 1968–1978 changes in heart, stroke, and cancer mortality.) In the midst of good news for all other leading causes of death, this is an important piece of bad news.

Older women and men die from the same problems. The top three causes of death for both sexes are heart disease, cancer, and cerebrovascular disease (stroke). These account for about three-fourths of women's death at ages 65 to 74, 75 to 84, and 85+ (Table 4.3); the same is true for men. Compared to men, larger percentages of women die from diabetes, stroke, and arteriosclerosis; smaller percentages from influenza/pneumonia, accidents, bronchitis/emphysema/asthma, cirrhosis, nephritis/nephrosis, and other artery diseases; and similar percentages from heart disease and cancer.

The cause-specific data are for underlying causes of death (the most significant health problem a person has at time of death). Death certificates also list other contributing and immediate causes. For example, the underlying cause may be chronic heart disease, with diabetes as a contributing cause and pneumonia as an immediate cause. Recently, researchers have been studying all of the causes listed to determine how often people die from several causes rather than just one, and to compute the prevalence of diseases before death (regardless of their position on the certificate). Three results are pertinent here: First, female decedents are more likely to have *several causes of death* than male decedents. In 1969, 60.7 percent of white female deaths had 2 or more causes, compared to 53.4 percent of white male deaths (Manton, 1980). A similar situation occurs for blacks (48.7% for black females, 40.2% for black males). (Note that these percentages are for all ages, not just older people.) Second, arteriosclerosis is often

Table 4.3
Leading Causes of Death for Older Women, United States, 1978

	Percent of All Deaths and Rank Among the Top Ten Causes					
	Ages 65–74		Ages 75–84		Ages 85+	
	Percent	Rank	Percent	Rank	Percent	Rank
Diseases of heart	38.5	1	45.5	1	49.3	1
Malignant neoplasms	27.5	2	16.4	2	8.4	3
Cerebrovascular diseases	9.7	3	14.8	3	17.0	2
Diabetes mellitus	3.0	4	2.6	5	1.6	7
Influenza/pneumonia	2.0	5	3.3	4	5.3	4
Accidents	1.9	6	1.7	7	1.8	6
Other diseases of arteries, arterioles, and capillaries[a]	1.4	7	1.4	8	1.5	8
Cirrhosis of liver	1.2	8	—[b]	—	—	—
Bronchitis/emphysema/ asthma	1.1	9	0.6	9	—	—
Arteriosclerosis	0.9	10	2.3	6	4.7	5
Nephritis/nephrosis	—	—	0.4	10	—	—
Hernia	—	—	—	—	0.4	9
Hypertension	—	—	—	—	0.4	10
All other causes	12.8		11.0		9.6	
Total	100.0		100.0		100.0	

Source: Unpublished tables from the National Center for Health Statistics.
[a]In vital statistics publications, this collection of diseases is usually excluded from "leading causes" lists. Because death rates for the category are relatively high among older persons, we choose to include it here.
[b]Not among the top ten causes of death for this age group.

present but not the primary cause of death. For underlying causes, it ranks fourth or fifth for people 75+ (Manton, 1980). But when all mentions are considered, it becomes the second-ranked cause of death for white men and women 75+, and third for black men and women. This new analysis shows that the three *leading causes* of death are all circulatory problems (ischemic heart disease, arteriosclerosis, stroke), and cancer moves to fourth or fifth place. Third, in this analysis, mortality rates rise for most diseases and by about the same magnitude for women and men. Thus, the *relative risks* of death for the sexes remain the same as in underlying cause data.

To sum up: Older women have had a longevity advantage over older men throughout this century. Women's rates dropped faster than men's, so their longevity advantage increased. Even in the 1950s, when older men's rates were at a standstill, older women's continued to fall a little. This situation of lower female rates and increasing sex differences occurred at all other ages, too. These trends cannot continue indefinitely; there are limits to mortality rates and human life span. In fact, the recent mortality declines are more similar for older women and men than the declines of earlier decades; so although the gap continues to widen, it does so more slowly than before (see Verbrugge, 1980).

As a direct result of these mortality trends, the older population is largely women. For ages 65 and over, there are 68 men per 100 women; for ages 85+, 45 men per 100 women. These sex ratios will continue to widen in the next 50 years, but not as fast as during the past 50 years. This is an important point: Population aging has been a prominent feature of the twentieth century. In our lifetimes, we have felt the rapid increase of older persons, especially older women, and we are in the midst of cultural and programmatic reactions. But most of the population aging and feminizing-of-the-elderly that the U.S. will experience has already occurred. Youngsters born in the 1970s and 1980s will find an old population already there, and they will not experience the dramatic increase we did.

PHYSICAL HEALTH OF OLDER WOMEN

The quality of life is as important as its quantity. Increasing a population's life expectancy is a fine achievement, but a compromised one if it means many years of symptoms and disability for older people (see Gruenberg, 1977). How older people feel on a daily basis, how prevalent chronic diseases are among them, and how much their social and physical activities are hampered by health problems are now key concerns of health researchers and health planners.

In this section, we present a profile of older women's health status and disability. The data come from health interviews with older women and from medical records.[3] The profile is con-

---

[3] The indicators reflect "poor health" rather than "good health." This is a common feature of health statistics, and it can cause an exaggerated impression of morbidity for the elderly, many of whom have no serious diseases and no limitations. Riley (1981b) recommends positive views of older people, and we hope that future health surveys will contain more items that emphasize wellness.

temporary, reflecting health in the 1970s and 1980s. Trends in health for older women and men are discussed elsewhere (Verbrugge, 1983a, 1983b).

General Health Status

About 9 percent of older women consider their health "poor," and 22 percent rate it as "fair" (National Center for Health Statistics, 1978a). On the positive side, 29 percent and 40 percent report "excellent" and "good" health, respectively. Older men are very similar in their evaluations, with a 9 percent "poor" and 23 percent "fair." But this similarity masks very different kinds of diseases and symptoms for the sexes, as the next sections will reveal.

Daily Health

There is very little information about daily discomforts and symptoms that elderly people (or any other age-group) feel. A 1957 national study asked older people to name health troubles experienced in the past four weeks. The leading problems for women were "general" discomforts (not associated with any specific condition), followed by circulatory disease symptoms, digestive symptoms, and musculoskeletal symptoms, in that order (Shanas, 1962). For older men, "general" discomforts also ranked first, followed by circulatory, ear, and musculoskeletal symptoms. In a 1978 Detroit study, respondents recorded daily symptoms for six weeks (Verbrugge, 1979). For older women and men, musculoskeletal problems were most frequent, followed by respiratory, general, and eye/ear symptoms for women; and by general, skin/nails/hair, and respiratory symptoms for men. We suspect that a current national survey would show rankings more like the Detroit survey than like the 1957 one. In sum, daily life for the elderly has many ill-defined aches and pains, as well as symptoms of specific chronic diseases such as arthritis, heart disease, emphysema/asthma, and cataract.

Acute Conditions and
Short-term Disability

Older people have acute illnesses (such as infections, colds, stomach upsets) less often than middle-aged people, but the ones that occur are more debilitating for them and require more care. Lower physical resistance and weaker recuperative capacities may account for this.

Older women have more frequent acute illnesses than do older men, and they average more days of bed rest for each illness (Table 4.4). This may indicate that women's illnesses are more severe, but it can also reflect women's greater concern to take curative actions when ill. Older men opt to reduce their activities partially, without going to bed. [The data sometimes show more total (bed + non-bed) restricted activity days per condition for men, yet fewer bed days; thus, more of them are non-bed.]

Each year, about 20 percent of older women suffer an injury that requires medical care or restricted activity (Metropolitan Life Foundation, 1982). Their injury rates are higher than older men's; this is a notable change from younger ages, when men's rates are higher. The majority of older women's injuries occur at home, compared to half of men's. Injuries are less frequent than respiratory illnesses, but they cause more restricted activity per occurrence. Injured older women have more days in bed than injured men, but a similar or fewer number of non-bed days. Again, this can reflect more serious injuries among the women or their greater propensity to take curative actions.

In sum: Older women suffer more acute illnesses and injuries than older men. They also have more bed disability for each illness and injury, but whether the reason is medical (more severe conditions) or psychosocial (belief in benefits of bed rest) is not known).

Chronic Conditions and
Long-term Disability

Data on the leading chronic conditions for older women and older men come from three different surveys, yet they point to the same key health problems. It should be noted that these data are based on self-reports of survey respondents.

Table 4.4
Acute Conditions and Short-term Disability for Older Women
and Older Men, United States[a]

	Women 65+	Men 65+
	(Rates are per 100 persons per year)	
Acute Conditions (1980)		
Incidence of acute conditions (rate)	126	97
Infective and parasitic diseases	8	7
Respiratory conditions	67	51
Digestive system conditions	7	—[b]
Injuries	22	14
All other acute conditions[c]	22	—
Average days of restricted activity per condition	9.4	9.1
Average days of bed disability per condition	3.9	3.4
Injuries (1978)		
Percent injured per year	26.0	16.1
Moving motor vehicle	1.5[d]	2.6[d]
At work	0.9[d]	—[e]
At home	16.0	8.0
Other	7.0	6.1[d]
Average days of restricted activity per injured person[f]	31.8	25.6
Average days of bed disability per injured person[f]	7.4	7.3

Sources: For Acute Conditions: Tabulations from the 1980 National Health Interview Survey prepared for the Metropolitan Life Foundation. *Statistical Bulletin*, 63, 1982. (Annual reports from the National Center for Health Statistics show age-sex specific rates for All Acute Conditions but not for the five categories.) For Injuries: Data from the 1978 National Health Interview Survey published in National Center for Health Statistics. *Vital and Health Statistics.* Series 10, No. 130. Hyattsville, Md., 1979b.
[a]Acute conditions are counted if they cause restricted activity or medical attention.
[b]Figures not available in source document.
[c]Examples are ear diseases, headaches, genitourinary disorders, and skin diseases which last less than three months.
[d]Figure is unreliable because of high sampling variability.
[e]No persons reported work injuries in this age-sex group in the 1978 survey.
[f]This is the average number of days of injury-related disability for people who suffered injury; this can cover several injury episodes. It is not the average days of disability per injury.

For older women, (1) *arthritis* stands out clearly as the most common condition. Fifty-three percent (53%) say they have diagnosed arthritis; a similar percent (45%) report arthritis in the past year. Arthritis persistently limits activities for 13 percent of older women. (2) *High blood pressure* ranks second in importance; about one-third of older women have it (34% in one survey, 24% in another). It is less disabling than arthritis; only 5 percent of older women say they limit housework or jobs because of it. (3) Eight percent (8%) report a heart attack in their lifetime, and 20 percent report current *heart conditions.* Heart disease often requires changes in daily life, and 10 percent of the women report limitations from it. (4) Other *musculoskeletal and circulatory problems* also bother older women: About 9 percent have leg or hip impairments; 12 percent, varicose veins; 14 percent, corns and callosities; and 8 percent, hemorrhoids. The leg and hip problems cause some major restrictions (3%); the other conditions seldom cause them. (5) Sensory problems are very prevalent; 22 percent of older women report *visual impairments* and 26 percent, *hearing impairments.* Of the two, visual problems are more severe: Even with corrective care such as glasses, 5 percent of older women report serious trouble seeing things. By contrast, only 1 percent report limitations due to deafness or hearing loss. (6) Nine percent (9%) report having *diabetes,* and it limits activities for 3 percent. (7) *Chronic respiratory conditions* (diseases and allergies) are quite common, but they seldom cause limitations for older women. In sum, the leading health problems reported by older women are musculoskeletal, circulatory, and respiratory conditions, and diabetes. Diseases of the skin and of the nervous, urinary, and digestive systems tend to rank lower in prevalence and limitations.

Comparing older men with older women: (1) Men are about half as likely to indicate the presence of arthritis (33% in one survey, 29% in the other) or be limited by it (8%). They report much less arthritis pain, swelling, and stiffness (Maurer, 1979). The most common site of arthritis is the knees for both sexes, but women's cases are especially concentrated there. Although arthritis is a very common chronic condition for older men, it does not stand out so strikingly for them as for women. (2) Heart disease is men's second ranking disease. More men (14%) than women have suffered a heart attack, and more (13%) have limitations due to heart disease. Men also have more stroke history and limitations from stroke. Overall, they have more cardiovascular problems of all kinds, except high blood pressure. (3) Men report more hearing impairments than women do, and they are more limited by them. By contrast, visual impairments are slightly less prevalent and limiting for men than for women; this will be buttressed by medical data in the next section. (4) Men are more likely to have serious respiratory diseases and to be limited by them. Chronic bronchitis, emphysema, and asthma appear more often for men and routinely rank higher for them. On the other hand, allergies of all kinds are less common for older men than for older women.

Some overall comments about prevalence rates for older people are in order: First, in each of the surveys, the top five conditions are the same for men and women (with one small exception). But the rank orders differ: Arthritis, hypertension, and allergies rank higher for women. Heart disease, respiratory disease, and hearing impairments rank higher for men. Second, hypertension and hearing impairments are very prevalent for older people, but they do not cause much long-term disability. By contrast, heart disease, orthopedic impairments, and cerebrovascular disease are especially likely to cause major restrictions. Third, several leading causes of death are not very prevalent as chronic conditions, but they are very life-threatening when they do occur. Malignant neoplasms, cerebrovascular disease (stroke), asthma, and arteriosclerosis seldom appear in self-reports. Rates for these are higher for men than for women and larger percentages of men are limited by the conditions.

Medical examinations were conducted during the National Health and Nutrition Examination Survey (1971–1974) and its predecessor the National Health Examination Survey (1960–1962).[4] The results concur with older people's self-reports of chronic problems. As shown in the more recent (1971–1974) survey, 25 percent of older women ages 65 to 74 have osteoarthritis of knees and 7 percent have "moderate or severe" cases as judged by clinicians (Table 4.5). One-third (36%) have definite hypertension, and another third (33%) have borderline hypertension. Forty-one percent (41%) have elevated serum cholesterol (260 mg/100 ml or higher); this is a risk factor for circulatory diseases.

Compared to men ages 65 to 74, women are more likely to have severe arthritis, high blood pressure, and elevated cholesterol. They have more vision dysfunctions, but less hearing loss and less skin pathology. They show more signs of previous dental work; this may partly explain their better current dental health (less periodontal disease or other clinical signs of dental needs).

---

[4]Data from the second National Health and Nutrition Examination Survey (1976–1980) are not yet available.

Table 4.5
Prevalence of Chronic Conditions and Risk Factors for Chronic Disease
Among Older Women and Older Men, Based on Medical
Examinations, United States

	Women 65–74	Men 65–74
	%	%
Arthritis		
Osteoarthritis of knees	24.9	13.7
Moderate or severe	6.6	2.0
Osteoarthritis of hips	3.1	6.2
Moderate or severe	1.2	2.3
Sacroiliitis	2.1	2.0
Moderate or severe	0.4	0.6
Hypertension		
Definite hypertension	36.0	31.8
Borderline hypertension	32.8	29.8
Cholesterol		
260 mg/100 ml or higher	40.7	20.9
Vision		
Poor distance vision (20/50 or worse in better eye, with usual correction)	14.5	13.5
Hearing		
Can hear and understand everyday speech at 20dB amplification	36.6	28.9
Skin		
Significant skin pathology	36.6	46.8
Needs care ("not now under best care")	8.5	11.6
Dental		
One arch edentulous	15.3	15.5
Both arches edentulous	47.0	43.6
Has periodontal disease	56.8	72.8
Has one or more specific dental needs (determined by examination)	55.5	68.2

Source: Data from the National Health and Nutrition Examination Survey I (1971–1974) published in National Center for Health Statistics. *Vital and Health Statistics.* Series 11, Nos. 201 (1977); 205; 212 (1978c,d); 213; 214 (1979c,d); 215 (1980c); and 221 (1981a).

Treated Conditions. Ambulatory care for older women focuses on their musculoskeletal aches and pain, acute respiratory illnesses, cardiovascular diseases, and vision problems, so they are less prominent as reasons for ambulatory care (Table 4.6) than in reported prevalence rates. Otherwise, the list of complaints that older women often bring to physicians mirrors the list of most prevalent conditions. But notice the prominence of circulatory diagnoses given by physicians; these emerge from a wide variety of complaints, which patients often attribute to noncirculatory problems. In terms of specific diagnoses, the most common conditions seen by physicians are high blood pressure, heart disease, and diabetes.

Hospitalization is prompted by life-threatening diseases and serious injuries. Here, the array of conditions is quite different from daily symptoms and office visits. The leading causes of hospital stays for older women are heart disease, cancer, fractures, and stroke (Table 4.6).

Similar shifts appear for older men, and some are quite striking. Although men seldom complain of cardiovascular symptoms, this is the main diagnosis given to them for office visits. Respiratory problems (some certainly chronic) are more prominent in ambulatory care for men than they are for women, but musculoskeletal and eye/ear problems are less prominent. Genitourinary (mainly prostate) conditions are more common for men, and they lead to hospital stays more often. Men's lower hospital rates for fractures may be due to two factors: Fall injuries are less common for older men than for older women (Hogue, 1982); and women's falls may result in fractures more often than men's falls do because of osteoporosis among women.[5]

From Daily Life to Death. It is fascinating to compare daily symptoms, prevalent conditions, treated conditions, and causes of death. Musculoskeletal and sensory problems are important in daily life for older women, but they seldom cause hospitalization or death. Cardiovascular problems are common at all stages, but there is a shift from hypertension (a risk factor) to heart failure itself. Reflecting its early asymptomatic nature and rapid course, cancer scarcely appears in the array of daily or ambulatory care problems, but it is a prominent cause of hospitalization and death.[6] Similarly, influenza and pneumonia are acute conditions

---

[5] Detailed tables of reported chronic conditions of elderly men and women are available from the author.

[6] Sex differences in cancer data are especially interesting: Older women report more current and past cancer. But older men are hospitalized more for it and have higher cancer mortality rates. In addition, a national surveillance program shows higher cancer incidence rates for men, for all types of malignancies except breast and endocrine (National Cancer Institute, 1981). The data reflect women's higher incidence of benign cancers (National Cancer Institute, 1981), possibly earlier diagnosis and treatment of malignant ones, and better prognosis for the types of malignancies they develop.

Table 4.6
Leading Complaints and Diagnoses for Ambulatory Care Visits and Leading Diagnoses for Hospital Discharges, Among Older Women and Older Men, United States

Principal complaints for office visits (general types) (Percent of symptomatic visits)a	Principal diagnoses for office visits (general types) (Percent of "sick" visits)b	Principal specific diagnoses for office visits (Percent of all visits)b	Principal specific diagnoses for hospital discharges (Discharges per 100,000 pop.)d
		Women 65+	
Muscle bone, 22.6	Circulatory, 25.0	Hypertension,g 11.0	Ischemic heart disease, 41.3
Respiratory, 15.7	Musculoskeletal, 12.4	Chronic ischemic heart disease, 6.1	Malignant neoplasms, 27.4
Digestive, 12.7	Nervous system/sense organs,f 10.2	Diabetes mellitus, 4.0	Fractures, all sites 20.6
Cardiovascular, 8.9	Respiratory, 8.5	Osteoarthritis and allied conditions, 3.3	Cerebrovascular disease, 19.6
Eyes/ears, 8.0	Endocrine/nutritional/metabolic, 6.8	Cataract, 3.0	Cataract, 11.7
General,e 7.8	Digestive, 5.9	Arthritis, unspecified, 2.1	Diabetes mellitus, 10.6
Genitourinary, 7.0	Genitourinary, 5.7	Symptomatic heart disease, 1.8	Arthritis/rheumatism, 10.1
Nervous, 7.0	Accidents/poisoning/violence, 5.1	Other diseases of eye,g 1.7	Pneumonia, all forms, 9.9
		Men 65+	
Muscle/bone, 21.5	Circulatory, 28.2	(Not available)	Ischemic heart disease, 51.9
Respiratory, 20.3	Respiratory, 12.0		Malignant neoplasms, 42.8
Digestive, 11.0	Nervous system/sense organs, 9.4		Cerebrovascular disease, 21.1
Skin/hair, 8.6	Muscle/bone, 7.9		Hyperplasia of prostate, 17.8
Genitourinary, 8.3	Endocrine/nutritional/metabolic, 6.9		Pneumonia, all forms, 13.1
General, 7.8	Genitourinary, 6.5		Congestive heart failure, 9.7
Eyes/ears, 7.4	Neoplasms, 5.6		Fractures, all sites, 9.7
Cardiovascular, 6.8	Accidents/poisoning/violence, 5.4		Cataract, 9.4

Sources: For principal complaints (general types) and principal diagnoses (general types): Unpublished data for the 1975 National Ambulatory Medical Care Survey. For information about the survey, see National Center for Health Statistics. *Vital and Health Statistics.* Series 13, No. 33. Hyattsville, Md., 1978e. For principal specific diagnoses for office visits: Data from the 1978 National Ambulatory Medical Care Survey, published in National Center for Health Statistics. *Vital and Health Statistics.* Series 13, No. 59. Hyattsville, Md., 1981b. For hospital discharges: Data from the 1975 National Hospital Discharge Survey, published in National Center for Health Statistics. *Vital and Health Statistics.* Series 13, No. 35. Hyattsville, Md., 1978f.

aThere are 13 general types of complaints (12 are for symptoms in different body sites, 1 is for all nonsymptomatic visits). Up to 3 complaints may be coded for a visit. The percentages here refer to the principal (first-listed) complaint and are based on symptomatic visits (thus, nonsymptomatic ones are excluded). For details about the symptom classification used for the 1975 survey, see National Center for Health Statistics (1974). *Vital and Health Statistics.* Series 2, No. 63. Hyattsville, Md. (The classification has been revised since then.)

bDiagnoses are coded according to the International Classification of Diseases (ICD-8), which has 18 general categories (17 are for illness and injury diagnoses, 1 is for exams/surgical aftercare/other nonsick visits). Up to 3 diagnoses may be coded for a visit. The percentages here refer to the principal (first-listed) diagnosis and are based on "sick" visits (those with an illness/injury diagnosis). For details about the ICD-8, see National Center for Health Statistics (1967). *Eighth Revision International Classification of Diseases.* USPHS Pub. No. 1693.

cThe ICD-8 has several hundred specific diagnosis codes. The table shows the most common specific illness/injury diagnoses (3-digit codes). The percentages here refer to all visits, whether "sick" or "nonsick."

dPatients can be alive or dead at time of discharge in this survey. Several diagnoses may be involved in a hospital stay; the percentages here refer to the principal diagnosis.

eExamples are chills, fatigue, fluid imbalance, weight gain, and generalized pain.

fExamples are multiple sclerosis, epilepsy, migraine, neuralgia/neuritis, and sciatica.

gThe ICD-8 title is essential benign hypertension (code 401).

seldom present in daily life, but they are very life-threatening for older women when they occur. Diabetes is the most consistent disease across stages, with moderate prevalence, treatment, and mortality rates.

Daily life for older women has many aches and pains that are bothersome but not life-threatening. Ultimately the "killer" conditions of heart disease, cancer, and stroke do manifest themselves and lead to death. By contrast, older men tend to be more bothered in daily life by precisely the problems (circulatory and respiratory) that cause their deaths. There is less difference across their lists of daily symptoms and prevalent conditions, and in treated conditions or causes of death, than for older women.

Overall, older women have more chronic health problems than men do (see Verbrugge, 1982b: Table 6). Their rates are higher for hypertension, arthritis, diabetes, anemia, migraine, sciatica, hypertensive disease, varicose veins, most digestive and urinary problems (except ulcer and hernia), allergies, and most orthopedic problems. These conditions are frequently symptomatic but not often fatal. By contrast, the list of conditions with higher male rates is shorter, and it contains most of the leading causes of death for older people (heart disease, cerebrovascular disease, arteriosclerosis, pneumonia, emphysema/asthma). Second, an early National Health Interview Survey (1957–1958) showed that 34 percent of older women had 3+ chronic ailments in contrast to 28 percent of older men (Public Health Survey, 1959). More recent Health Interview Survey data are not available. Third, we noted earlier that female decedents have more causes listed on their death certificates than male decedents. This may partly be due to women's older ages at death, which gives them more time to accumulate serious health problems.

Social, Physical, and Mobility Limitations. Overall, 35 percent of older women say they are limited in their major activity (housework or job) by a chronic conditions (Table 4.7). An additional 8 percent say they have limitations only in secondary activities like church, clubs, and social events. More often than older men, older women have trouble in physical activities like climbing stairs and lifting objects, and in personal care activities like bathing and eating. They have more mobility problems too; 6 percent report trouble getting around alone, another 7 percent need help in getting around, and 5 percent are confined to home. The total mobility problem is 19 percent, compared to 15 percent for men. More older women use aids such as canes, special

Table 4.7
Chronic Conditions and Long-term Disability for Older Women
and Older Men, United States

	Women 65+ (%)	Men 65+ (%)
Limitations of activity due to chronic condition (1978)		
Limited in major activity	34.9	43.2
Limited but not in major activity	7.8	5.0
Difficulty in doing common tasks (1962)		
Walking up and down stairs	35	24
Getting around the house	8	4
Washing/bathing	13	7
Dressing/putting on shoes	9	7
Cutting toenails	22	15
Limitation of mobility due to chronic condition (1972)		
Has trouble getting around alone	6.1	5.4
Needs help in getting around	7.2	6.0
Confined to house	5.4	4.9
Disability days for chronic conditions (1977)[a]	Averages (days per person per year)	
Restricted activity days (bed + nonbed)	27.6 days	22.8 days
Bed disability days	11.2 days	8.2

Sources: For limitation and disability days: National Center for Health Statistics. *Vital and Health Statistics,* Series 10, Nos. 96 (1974), 126 (1978b), 130 (1979b). For common tasks see: Shanas, E. et al. *Old People in Three Industrial Societies.* New York: Atherton Press, 1968.
[a]Estimated from Total disability days (1977) minus disability days for acute conditions (July 1977–June 1978).

shoes, walkers, and wheelchairs (Black, 1980), but more older men have artificial limbs or use braces. Each year, older women average about 28 days of restricted activity for chronic problems; 11 of those are spent in bed. For older men, the comparable figures are 23 days and 8 days. (For data on how joint conditions limit women and men, see Maurer, 1979. Disability data from a community survey are reported in Branch and Jette, 1981; Jette and Branch, 1981.)

In sum: Virtually all disability statistics show older women more limited than older men. This may be a function in part of the disproportionate number of very old women among those aged 65 and above. It also reflects the kinds of health problems women have (often musculoskeletal), their severity (more serious musculoskeletal ones), and women's caretaking behavior. There is one persistent exception: A larger percentage of older men say they have problems in their "main activity" because of a chronic condition. It is difficult to interpret this because older men are asked about problems in having a paid job, whereas most older women are asked about housework. A given health problem is more likely to limit job activity than housework, and this certainly boosts men's reports of limitation. Thus, men's responses may reflect physical demands of jobs (compared to housework) more than the prevalence or severity of their chronic conditions.

A Summary of Health

Older women are bothered by chronic problems more than older men are, largely because the kinds of conditions they have differ. Women specialize in conditions that are frequently symptomatic and cause partial limitations but are not life-threatening. Men specialize in fatal conditions. In one sense, older women have poorer health status than older men because their daily lives are more troubled by symptoms (acute and chronic) and because they find it more difficult to perform social, physical, and mobility activities. In another sense, older men have poorer health, but this is less visible since they have fewer daily symptoms and possibly less diagnosis and treatment before death.

LINKS BETWEEN MORBIDITY AND MORTALITY

The health profile of older women is quite different from their death profile. The basic reason is that women's typical symptoms are from "nonkiller" conditions; that is, diseases that seldome cause death. Ultimately women die from the same diseases as men do, but at later ages. The delay allows them to accumulate nonkiller conditions that often cause more daily bother than any "killer" conditions they have.

Why are prevalence rates for life-threatening conditions lower for women? Four explanations are possible: First, females may have greater biological resistance to most cardiovascular diseases and possibly to malignant neoplasms. Second, during life, women's roles may give them less exposure to the causative agents of heart disease, cancer, and stroke. For example, employed women usually have less exposure to noxious chemicals than employed men do. In addition, women may respond to those agents in less health-damaging ways. For example, they may vent job upsets with friends and family, whereas men remain silent and internalize the stress. This is a capsule statement for many specific hypotheses about risk factors, sex differences in those factors, and the etiological link between risk factors and particular chronic conditions. Third, women probably have their chronic conditions diagnosed earlier and treatment initiated earlier than men do. If so, women slow the progress of their chronic diseases. By contrast, when men's conditions are diagnosed, it may often be too late for effective medical intervention. Fourth, women's personal health practices throughout life may also help them. Years of paying more attention to illness (such as more bed rest) and more preventive actions (such as vitamin use) may actually give them greater resistance in their older ages. What counts as poor health in the short run might promote good health in the long-run. These four explanations are discussed in more detail elsewhere (Verbrugge, 1982a). Scientific evidence on them is accumulating and generally supports the statements above (see Belloc, 1973; Belloc & Breslow, 1972; Berkman, 1975; Berkman & Syme, 1979; Mossey & Shapiro, 1982; Palmore, 1969a, 1969b; Pfeiffer, 1970; Waldron, 1976, 1982; Wiley & Camacho, 1980; Wingard, 1982; Wingard, Suarez, & Barrett-Connor, 1983). We may never fully know the relative importance of biology, role, medical care, and health habit factors in women's longevity advantage; and their importance may change over time as adults' roles, health care practices, and health attitudes change.

Why are prevalence rates for nonkiller conditions higher for women? Two explanations are plausible: First, females may be more biologically vulnerable to bone and joint deterioration, eye diseases and vision loss, and hypertension. Second, by living longer, women have more chance to "wear out." Musculoskeletal and sensory problems increase with age for virtually all persons, and they may be natural companions of the aging body. Within any age grouping (such as 65–69), women tend to predominate, so their chances of having musculoskeletal and sensory problems are greater. Health statistics can seldom take this into account adequately. These two explanations are biological and artifactual ones. They are speculative, and scientific evidence on them is incomplete. Hypotheses about roles, medical care, and health habits are not stated here; but it is hard to see how women's behaviors in these areas would increase their risks of developing non-killer conditions over men's risks.

THE FUTURE HEALTH PROFILE
OF OLDER WOMEN

For most of the twentieth century, public health efforts have been aimed at reducing mortality rates so that individuals live more years. Mortality rates are now low; although they may continue to drop for some diseases, this will not increase life expectancy much because survivors of one disease become exposed to other life-threatening ones (Keyfitz, 1977, 1978; Tsai, Lee, & Hardy, 1978). Public health attention is therefore turning toward the quality of life rather than its length. The goal is to help individuals maintain vigor and good physical functioning; in other words, to postpone disability as well as death (see U.S. Department of Health, Education and Welfare, 1979).

Public policy and regulations alone cannot realize this goal. Individuals must also have health attitudes and habits that minimize their risks of serious illness and injury. In the 1970s and 1980s, the importance of individual responsibility for health is being emphasized (Knowles, 1977), and adults are devoting more time and attention to diet, exercise, moderation of smoking and drinking, and stress reduction.

Changes like these make it very difficult to predict the health of future cohorts of older women, compared to contemporary ones. When they reach their 60s and 70s, the coming cohorts will have had lifetimes that differ greatly from current cohorts. For example, more women will have long employment experience, a divorce sometime during life, prolonged stresses and satisfactions from multiple roles (wife, mother, and worker). They will have had more years of modern medical care, including use of therapeutic and preventive drugs, and also prompt hospital care for illness. And they will probably have made more personal investment in their health through attentive health habits and lifestyles. Moreover, medical care may be even more effective than now, so that diseases are arrested more completely and sometimes even cured. All of these changes bode well for the health of women who will be elderly in future decades.

This is a likely health profile for future cohorts: First, older women will *feel better* on a daily basis. Symptoms will be alleviated more easily because of better drugs and other therapy for chronic diseases, and because of better health habits during old and earlier ages. More healthful lifetimes should actually reduce the chances of developing chronic diseases, especially "killer" conditions. The kinds of problems older women have will probably shift toward "nonkiller" conditions (especially musculoskeletal and sensory ones), while "killer" conditions recede. Second, older women will have *fewer functional disabilities*, compared to women the same age today. They will be able to work and socialize more easily, lift and manipulate objects, climb stairs, perform personal care activities (bathing, dressing, cutting toenails, etc.), and move about freely at home and away. Again this will be the result of better medical care and better lifetime health habits. Third, older women will *live longer*. Those who reach age 65 can expect several more years of life than women who now reach 65. Greater longevity at older ages will be due to more healthful milieux and behaviors throughout life, and to better preventive and curative medical care. Fourth, the *death process will be shorter* and will involve the simultaneous breakdown of many body functions. In other words, severe morbidity will be compressed into a short time just before death, and "everything will fall apart at once." This compression of morbidity is possible if diseases are prevented or arrested better for future cohorts. For a compelling discussion of this phenomenon, see Fries (1980) and Fries and Crapo (1981); for a critique, see Manton (1982). In sum, older women will have longer lives that are more free of discomfort and disability.

This profile pertains to individuals. In other words, comparing a woman currently 75 years old with a woman that age in 2010, the future woman will probably feel better each day, have fewer disabilities, live longer, and die more rapidly. By contrast, if we ask about health for the whole population of older women, the profile may differ a bit. Improvements in mortality rates at older ages will increase the average age of the population 65+. Because health problems increase with age, statistics may sometimes show larger percentages of older people with symptoms, diseases, and limitations than now simply because a larger percentage of the population is very elderly. Thus, individual chances of good health may increase, although some population statistics can show worsening or no change—an artifact of age composition. Scientists and policymakers who watch health trends should be aware of this possibility.

What about the health of future older men? Men too will benefit from social, medical, and personal changes, so that future cohorts will change in the same directions as women.

Will older men and women differ in their health and mortality as much as now? We have noted many sex differences for contemporary older people; these will probably become smaller in the future but never completely disappear. The shift toward more similar health and mortality will come from changes made by both sexes in their roles, medical care behavior, and health habits. Higher labor force participation is exposing women to risks that were mainly felt by men in the past. It is speculated that cardiovascular disease rates will increase for women, but the truth is not yet known. On the other hand, men will probably improve their health habits and use more medical care in middle-age, so they become more similar to women in these respects. In general, the roles and habits of adult men and women may become more similar (but hopefully not identical) in coming decades. This means that morbidity and mortality risks will also become similar. Still, older women will probably continue to have more daily symptoms (especially musculoskeletal ones) and greater longevity, because of their different biological vulnerabilities and strengths.

Thus, we end with a positive view of future health for older women. The chances are that an older woman will have a more comfortable and active life than her same-age peer today. And a larger fraction of U.S. females will reach older ages and have the opportunity to enjoy healthful old age.

5
The Aging Skeleton

ROBERT LINDSAY

Loss of bone mass with age results eventually in a skeleton unable to withstand even trivial trauma. At this stage, recognized only when patients present to their physician with fracture, the diagnosis of osteoporosis is made. By that time point, however, the phenomenon of bone loss may have been progressing silently for some 10 to 20 years. The increasing incidence of osteoporosis and its insidious development have led to the use of the term "silent epidemic" to describe what is becoming an increasing public health problem. In this chapter we shall examine the epidemiology of the problem, the pathogenesis, prevention, and treatment of the disease and outline some possible future trends.

Since Albright's original work published about 40 years ago, it has been recognized that osteoporosis is predominantly a disease affecting the female of the species (Albright, Blomberg, & Smith, 1940). This is even more true today as the population over the age of 65 years continues to expand and to become even more predominantly female. The female:male ratio is now almost 2:1 for persons over 65 years. Recent evidence has suggested that the incidence of osteoporotic fractures may be increasing.

This trend is occurring as a result of both this increasing number of aged individuals in society and this increasing preponderance of females over males in the age-group 65 years and over. Additionally, however, there may be an age-independent increase in fracture incidence, the reason for which is as yet unknown. Since osteoporosis may be potentially a preventable condition, *it is doubly unfortunate that it is such a significant source of both morbidity and mortality.* Indeed, expenditures for hip fracture acute care alone may top $3.0 billion by the year 1990 and almost 50,000 individuals will die each year within three months of their fracture. Prediction from current data suggests that there may be 0.5 million hip fractures per year by the end of the century.

Recent advances in medical science have resulted in the availability of techniques that can detect bone loss at an early stage (Table 5.1). Since osteoporosis is a disease of bone mass with progressive loss of bone over a prolonged period of time, it would be most beneficial and perhaps also cost-effective if such bone loss could be prevented. The introduction of these sensitive techniques for determination of bone mass and bone loss has made the institution of preventive therapy a realistic possibility. Additionally, pharmacological agents that can retard bone loss are now available to physicians. Potentially, therefore, this disease is preventable. It is important to alert both health care professionals and the public, not only to these facts, but also to the risks and benefits of either instituting therapy during the silent phase of the disease or of delaying therapy until after fracture has occurred. We must also consider, therefore, the approaches to therapy that are available for those millions of women (estimated some 2–5 million) in the United States who now have evidence of the disease and may have become symptomatic. Such women usually have presented with one of three fractures: (1) fractures of the vertebral bodies, so-called crush fractures; (2) Colles' fractures, or fractures of the distal radius; and (3) fractures of the neck of the femur, or hip fractures. While both Colles' fractures and fractures of the vertebral body may result in significant morbidity, a significant mortality (5–15%) follows fractures of the hip, and nearly one-third of all affected individuals will enter nursing homes as a direct result of their fractures.

Table 5.1
Methods of Measurement of Bone Technique

	Coefficient of Variation
Radiogrammetry	2 – 0%
Radiodensity	5 – 15%
Single Beam Photon Absorptiometry	2 – 5%
Dual Beam Photon Absorptiometry	2 – 5%
Comptom Scattering	Approx 5%
(Ultrasound)	?
Computerized Axial Tomography	1 – 2%
Bone-Biopsy—Quantitative Histology	5 – 15%

EPIDEMIOLOGY OF OSTEOPOROSIS

It is a well documented fact that fracture incidence increases with age. Indeed, studies have shown that the incidence of all fractures increases after the age of 45. However, the increment for the so-called osteoporotic group of fractures is significantly greater, and in addition the upward trend in fracture incidence occurs earlier and rises faster in women than it does in men (Garraway, Stauffer, Kurland, & O'Fallon, 1979) (Figure 5.1). It has been postulated that almost 1 in 4 women over age of 65 will have evidence of osteoporotic fractures and that almost 1 woman in 4 will have had a hip fracture before reaching the age of 80, with a significant proportion of these having suffered bilateral hip fractures.

Recent data from the United Kingdom indicate that there may be an increasing incidence of osteoporosis (A. F. Lewis, 1981). Data analyzed by our laboratory (Lindsay & Herrington, 1983) indicate that fractures of the neck of the femur and vertebral fractures are becoming more frequent in the United States as causes of hospital admission (Figures 5.2 and 5.3). Femoral neck fractures probably cost $1.4 billion per year in acute health care cost currently, and this figure will rise to $3 billion by the end of this decade (Figure 5.4). In addition, it has been estimated that 20,000 to 30,000 individuals will die within 3 months of the hip fracture in the United States this year and that a further 50,000 will require long-term care at a cost to the country of at least $1.5 billion per year.

The total health care cost for all services to all individuals as a result of osteoporotic fractures is currently incalculable. An estimate of overall population trends suggests that by the year 2000 there will be approximately 20 million women over age 65 and about 500,000 hip fractures per year, with perhaps 5 million women having evidence of clinical osteoporosis and vertebral crush fractures. Considerable interest is therefore being focused now on the early identification of those individuals who may be at risk in order that attempts may be made to prevent the disease during its early silent years.

THE PATHOGENESIS OF BONE LOSS

Cross-sectional studies in which bone mineral mass has been measured by non-invasive techniques have generally indicated that bone mass begins to fall in the population at about age 30 to 40

FIGURE 5.1   Incidence for all fractures in males and females as a function of age. Data from Rochester, Minnesota. (From Garraway, Stauffer, Kurland, & O'Fallon, 1979. Limb fractures in a defined population 1. Frequency and distribution. *Mayo Clinic Proceedings, 54,* 701–707. With permission.)

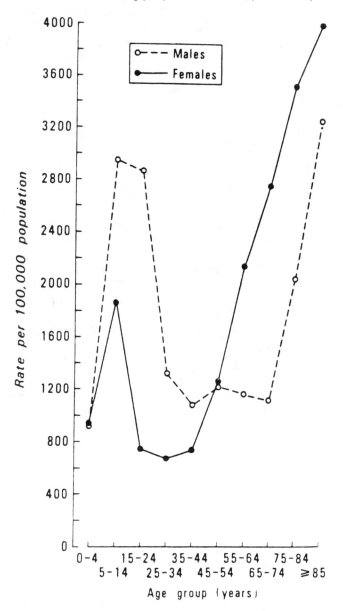

FIGURE 5.2   **Prevalence of hip fracture in the United States from 1970 through 1980.** Fractures are in thousands and data obtained from hospital admission data. (Commission on Professional and Hospital Activities data source.)

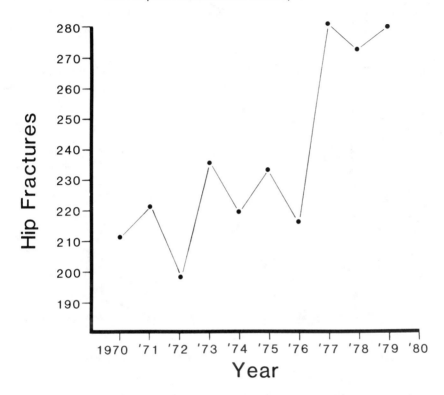

years of age. Women have less bone mass at maturity than men, and subsequently lose bone faster than men with an acceleration of bone loss occurring following the menopause, an outcome usually seen more clearly in longitudinal studies. The overall rate of bone loss appears to be about 1–2% per annum in the early years with increases in women to be between 1% and 3% of total skeletal mass per year following the menopause or oophorectomy (Lindsay & Hart, 1978). Although the role of the menopause in bone loss was described originally by Fuller Albright (Albright et al., 1940), the mechanisms by which the ovarian hormones affect bone are still not clearly understood.

Clearly, osteoporosis is a disease of multiple pathogenetic mechanisms, of which the menopause and subsequent loss of

FIGURE 5.3   **Prevalence of vertebral fractures in the United States from 1970 through 1980.** (Data obtained as in Figure 5.2.)

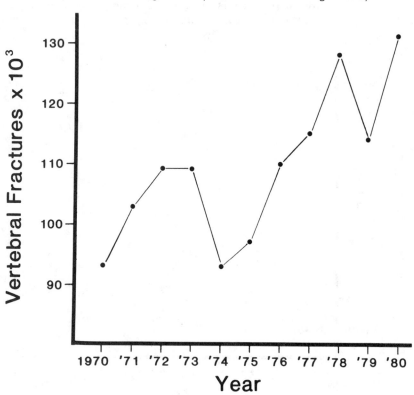

ovarian hormones is only one. It is a disease peculiarly associated with the white female and appears to be associated with a number of risk factors (Table 5.2). The identification of such risk factors

Table 5.2
Potential Risk Factors for Osteoporosis

White
Female
Low weight for height
Early menopause or oophorectomy
Family history of osteoporosis
Poor diet: Low calcium, high caffeine/alcohol
Sedentary lifestyle
Nulliparity

FIGURE 5.4   Estimated cost of acute health care for fractures of the neck
of the femur for the whole of the United States. Projections
for 1985 and 1990 are based on 5 percent annual inflation
rate, projected population increases (> 65 yrs.) and *no*
changes in physician or hospital reimbursement.

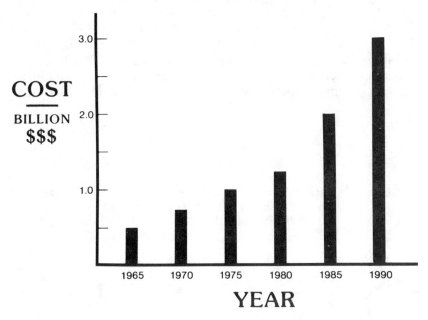

allows physicians a crude determination of patients who may be
at risk. However, the interaction of these risk factors and the
importance of their accumulation in a single individual has yet to
be analyzed.

The relative importance of dietary factors, which may be
most correctable when discovered at an early age, is to some
extent still unclear. However, recent evidence suggests that the
low-calcium diet characteristic of women in the United States
is a significant risk factor for this disease (Heaney, 1965). The
recommended daily intake of calcium is 800 mg per day and
most dietary studies have indicated that the average middle-aged
woman in the United States obtains only about 400 to 600 mg
per day in her diet (Avioli, 1981) (Figure 5.5). One study from
Yugoslavia (Matković et al., 1979) has indicated that there is
both higher bone mass and reduced fracture incidence in areas
where calcium intake is naturally high (800 to 1000 mg per

day) in comparison to villages with low calcium intake (Figure 5.6). It is, of cource, important to realize that exposure to a high-calcium diet in this study was lifelong, and we have no way of knowing whether or not changing calcium intake at a later age will significantly affect fracture incidence. However, from Heaney's data (Heaney, Recker, & Saville, 1978) it is clear that even in premenopausal women in North America the difference between intake and output results in a negative calcium balance of about 20 mg per day, resulting in an annual loss of about 7 grams of calcium per year, equating with the documented overall loss of approximately 1–2% of the total skeletal mass (Garra-

FIGURE 5.5 **Calcium intake of men and women in the United States as a function of age.** (From U.S. Department of Health, Education, and Welfare Publication No. HRA 77-1647, July 1977.)

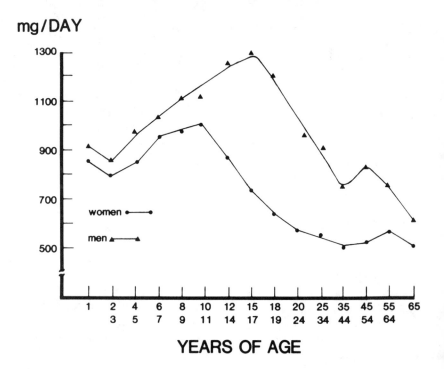

FIGURE 5.6   Fracture incidence as a function of life in two villages of Yugoslavia, one having lifetime high-calcium intake from natural sources, the other low. (Matković, Kostial, Simonovic, Buzina, Brodarec, & Nordin, 1979. Bone status and fracture rates in two regions of Yugoslavia. *American Journal of Clinical Nutrition, 32,* 540–549. With permission.)

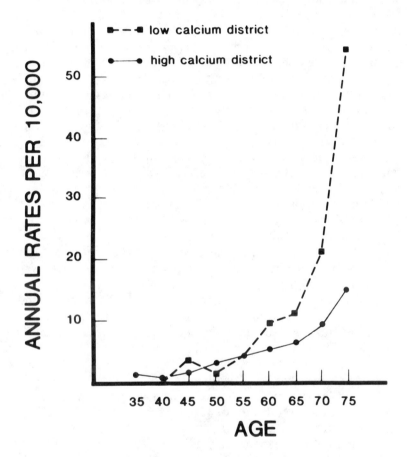

way et al., 1979). In the postmenopausal woman the difference between intake and output doubles, resulting in a negative calcium balance of approximately 40 mg per day or 13.6 grams per year, or a loss equivalent to the 1% to 2% reduction of total skeletal mass. Potentially, since there is normally a positive relationship between calcium intake and balance, raising calcium intake should correct this negative calcium balance. However, to reduce these relatively small deficits in calcium balance, large increments in dietary calcium are required, raising daily intake requirement to at least 1.5 g/day in postmenopausal women.

In addition, certain differences occur between the sexes in the endocrine systems controlling calcium and phosphate homeostasis, and these differences may have some importance in the pathogenesis of this disease. For example, several studies (Deftos et al., 1980; Hillyard, Stevenson, & MacIntyre, 1978) have not shown that the female is relatively calcitonin deficient in comparison to the male. The hormone calcitonin is an important inhibitor of bone resorption. Only during pregnancy or treatment with the oral contraceptives do calcitonin levels rise in women to approximate values found in men. In addition, in women the response of calcitonin to a normal stimulus appears to be limited in comparison to that occurring in men, and falls off even more rapidly with age. This discrepancy between circulating levels of calcitonin in males and females is exaggerated following the menopause. In postmenopausal females there is almost no rise in calcitonin following intravenous infusion of calcium (Deftos et al., 1980). It is tempting to speculate on whether such differences in endocrine status indicate why there is a difference in bone loss between men and women. However, such cause and effect has yet to be shown.

Undoubtedly, however, the relatively sudden loss of ovarian sex hormones at the climacteric contributes in a major fashion to the known loss of bone in women. In carefully designed studies it can be shown, not only that bone loss increases rapidly following the menopause, but that the subsequent rate of loss is somewhat dependent upon the remaining levels of sex steroids (Figure 5.7).

Certainly we know that women are more at risk for a number of reasons; as we have said, bone mass at maturity is lower in women and the overall rate of loss is greater. The relative importance of bone mass at maturity and the subsequent rate of loss in determining the increased fragility of the bone in older individuals has yet to be established. Currently we feel that to institute preventive measures, we must make techniques for measurement of bone mass available to a greater variety of physicians than before. Using procedures developed in our laboratory, we can now determine, within a 24-hour period, both bone mass and the current rate of loss of bone for any individual.

FIGURE 5.7   The relationship between circulating androstenedione and circulating estrogen levels in oophorectomized women. (●) indicates women losing bone at a relatively rapid rate, (▲) indicates those women losing bone slowly or not at all.

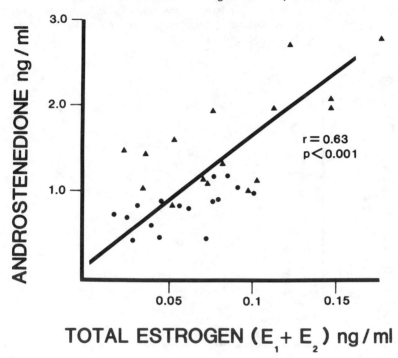

PREVENTION OF BONE LOSS

Over the past decade, several studies carried out in groups of young individuals using carefully controlled methods have indicated that bone loss may be prevented with appropriate pharmacological means.

Studies in our laboratory (Lindsay et al., 1976; Lindsay, Hart, Forrest, & Baird, 1980) have shown that estrogens effectively prevent bone loss in either oophorectomized or postmenopausal women (Figure 5.8). Treatment with estrogens appears to reduce bone resorption with a somewhat more delayed reduction in bone

FIGURE 5.8   **The effect of Mestranol (A) 24 μg/day (average daily dose)
on bone mineral content of oophorectomized women.** (P)
indicates those women treated with a placebo. Double-blind
controlled study of 120 women. (Lindsay, Hart, Aitken,
MacDonald, Anderson, & Clark, 1976. Long-term prevention of postmenopausal osteoporosis by oestrogens, *Lancet,
ii,* 1038–1040.)

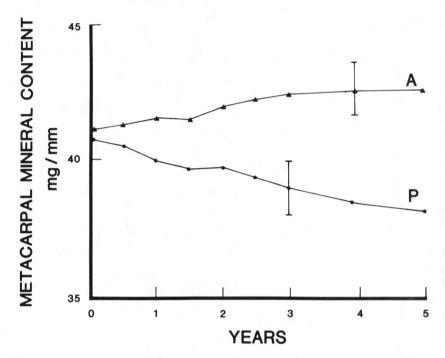

formation, since these two are intimately linked by poorly understood homeostatic mechanisms. The reduction in bone resorption,
however, appears greater than that which occurs in bone formation resulting in, for a short period at least, a positive bone balance and over a long period a reduced, if not abolished, negative
bone balance. Several studies have appeared in the literature over
the last decade confirming our results (Christiansen, Christiansen,

& Transbøl, 1981; Horsman, Gallagher, Simpson, & Nordin, 1977; Nachtigall, Nachtigall, Nachtigall, & Beckman, 1979; Recker, Saville, & Heaney, 1977).

More recently, we have looked at other compounds for their potential to protect against bone loss and have shown that all steroids that protect against bone loss effectively reduce bone turnover. Certain anabolic steroids (Lindsay, Hart, & Kraszewski, 1980) will do this and certain progestogens will also (Lindsay, Hart, Purdie, et al., 1978). Removal of the drug or termination of treatment results in the reintroduction of bone loss (Lindsay, Hart, MacLean, et al., 1978) at a rate consistent with reestablishment of the postmenopausal state. Recent studies have indicated that the minimum effective dose of the most commonly prescribed estrogen that must be given in order to prevent bone loss in most postmenopausal females is 0.625 mg per day of conjugated equine estrogens (Lindsay & Hart, 1982). Estrogens should be prescribed in a cyclical fashion to women with an intact uterus and a progestogen may be added into the therapy for the last ten days without any apparent detriment to the final effect on bone.

Our long-term study of the effect of estrogens has indicated that over a ten-year period oophorectomized women treated with placebo begin to show height loss whereas estrogen-treated women do not (Lindsay, Hart, Forrest, & Baird, 1980). Therefore, for the first time prospective data suggest that estrogens are protecting against bone structural failure. Retrospective and case control data have previously suggested protection against fracture by estrogen exposure of postmenopausal women (Hutchinson, Polansky, & Feinstein, 1979; Kreiger, Kelsey, Holford, & O'Connor, 1982).

As we have stated, several other laboratories have produced similar results, mostly in shorter term studies, and it is now clear that whenever estrogens are used for the prevention of bone loss, they are remarkably effective.

MODE OF ACTION OF ESTROGENS

Although all of these studies have been unanimous in indicating an effect of estrogen in prevention of bone loss, it is still somewhat unclear how estrogens exert their effect. Studies have failed to show estrogen receptors in bone and it has been suggested that estrogens must produce their effect on bone by an indirect mechanism involving perhaps the endocrine systems more usually associated with mineral homeostasis, the parathyroid hormone, vitamin D, calcitonin axis. If that is so, it is tempting to link estrogens to the relative calcitonin deficiency of women described above. Undoubtedly, estrogens either as oral contraceptives or when provided as therapy for postmenopausal women elevate circulating calcitonin levels (Hillyard et al., 1978). This rise in calcitonin could result in inhibition of bone resorption, the most significant biological effect of calcitonin. The inhibition of bone resorption would in turn result in a small fall in serum calcium, which would stimulate parathyroid hormone production. The rise in parathyroid hormone, by stimulating production of 1,25-dihydroxyvitamin D by the kidney, would increase the absorption of calcium from the diet. In addition, the small rise in parathyroid hormone could account for the reduction in calcium output in the urine (in addition to the reduced production of calcium from bone as a result of the decrement of bone resorption) and also the relative phosphate link that occurs in estrogen-treated women. The rise in 1,25-dihydroxyvitamin D could potentially increase bone resorption, but this may be prevented by the calcitonin increment. Such a thesis sounds nice, since it accounts for the major biochemical effects resulting from estrogen therapy. However, it is as yet still hypothetical. Large doses of calcitonin have been shown to increase total body calcium in osteoporotic individuals (Chestnut, Ivey, Nelp, & Baylink, 1979), but calcitonin that requires administration by subcutaneous or intramuscular injection has not as yet been used in the treatment of asymptomatic younger women for prevention of bone loss.

THE ROLE OF DIETARY
CALCIUM SUPPLEMENTATION

The possible importance of dietary calcium deficiency suggests that calcium supplementation may also be a useful mechanism for prevention of bone loss. Indeed, two short-term studies (Horsman et al., 1977; Recker et al., 1977) (two years in duration) have indicated that calcium supplementation may reduce bone loss. In both instances dietary supplementation of calcium was not as effective as estrogen therapy. However, these results do tend to support the argument that the recommended dietary intake of calcium is significantly low. Indeed, Heaney's work has suggested that premenopausal women require approximately 1000 mg per day calcium intake in order to maintain calcium balance. In postmenopausal women, the requirements for calcium appear to increase to approximately to 1.5 grams per day. Provision of this amount of calcium in the diet, therefore, for the average individual should result in a marked reduction in loss of mineral from the skeleton. The mechanism by which calcium does this is not likely to be the same as that of estrogens, however, since the biochemical effects of calcium supplementation are a small rise in serum calcium, reduction of parathyroid hormone, and an increase in urine calcium. Undoubtedly a reduction in bone turnover does occur since urine hydroxyproline is reduced. More investigation of the role of intervention with calcium supplements is still required, particularly if the effects of high calcium intake of a lifetime duration are confirmed to be as dramatic as reported by Matković (Matković et al., 1979).

TREATMENT OF THE ESTABLISHED DISEASE

Most therapeutic regimens that have been tried for the treatment of established disease have produced somewhat disappointing results. In the main, this is probably because we have in our current therapeutic armamentarium almost no agents that will stimulate bone formation and/or inhibit bone resorption without affecting bone formation and thereby increasing bone mass. Since the eventual requirement of therapy is primarily a reduction in the fragility of bone and its liability to fracture, such agents are required since the strength of bone is directly related to its mineral content. The pharmacological agents that reduce bone resorption will simply, by virtue of the homeostatic mechanisms linking resorption and formation, reduce both, and may prevent bone loss, but will almost never result in increase of bone mass of significant dimensions. However, two recent approaches have shown some promise. In the first study carried out at the Mayo Clinic, Riggs and his colleagues showed a significant reduction in fracture incidence in patients treated with multiple pharmacological agents (Riggs, Seeman, Hodgson, Taves, & O'Fallon, 1982). Once again, calcium supplementation and estrogen therapy appeared to be the mainstays of therapy. However, for maximum results, Riggs added sodium fluoride to the regimen with an apparent reduction in fracture incidence to about 10 percent of the untreated controls. Fluoride, which does stimulate osteoblast function and therefore bone formation, produces somewhat disorganized bone in comparison to the normal lamella on structure of adult bone. In addition, extra osseous bone formation tends to occur. In the second study, from Toronto (Harrison et al., 1981), somewhat similar results were produced. Significant increments in calcium in the lower third of the spine were obtained with a combination of estrogen and fluoride therapy. However, fluoride, which is converted to hydrofluoric acid in the stomach, is a toxin and in the Riggs study 38 percent of individuals suffered either gastrointestinal side effects or a fluoride arthropathy. The arthropathy tends to subside when therapy is discontinued. Gastrointestinal irritation, however, may result in hematemesis from ulceration and can be a potentially serious complication. Studies are underway currently to confirm this original Riggs observation and to determine the relative cost/benefit of the prescription of fluoride to the patients with established osteoporosis. Currently, fluoride is not recommended for the general treatment of osteoporosis, and it has not been cleared by the FDA for this use. Of major importance in the Mayo Clinic study was the indication that the addition of vitamin D to therapy appeared to be irrelevant and indeed unless we can demonstrate significant improvement in absorption of calcium by vitamin D, we do not routinely provide vitamin D as therapy for our patients.

Another exciting approach has been the use of low-dose parathyroid hormone therapy (Harrison et al., 1981), which appears to produce an anabolic effect in normal individuals and in osteoporotic patients. Increases in trabecular bone volume have been noted with improvement in calcium kinetic behavior. However, calcium balance does not appear to improve, perhaps suggesting a relocation of bone rather than the overall formation of new bone with an increase in total bone mass.

With our increasing capability to measure bone mass by noninvasive techniques, it does appear possible that we now have at long last the means by which to test the competence of therapeutic effects for osteoporosis even in the presence of established disease. However, it seems likely that this is one disorder in which prevention will remain significantly more effective than a cure.

THE ROLE OF EXERCISE

In addition to therapy using pharmacologic agents, it is clear that the progress of the disease may be influenced by advice of a more general variety. Individuals at risk and those with active disease should be encouraged to reduce cigarette smoking and alcohol consumption; limit their intake of caffeine; and participate in exercise programs to the limits of their capabilities. These all-around guides to general health are, in our Clinic, the starting point for both preventive therapy and treatment of established disease. Exercise programs must be designed *specifically* for each patient on an individual basis. While younger patients without overt crush fractures may be encouraged to walk or even run, if there are no other medical contraindications, greater caution is required when dealing with patients who have already fractured. During the immediate postfracture period, bed rest with adequate medication may be required for relief of pain. However, as soon as the patient can tolerate it, we encourage mobilization. Often at this stage a spinal support will allow earlier mobilization with less pain. However, we actively discourage the use of a support except for pain relief, and do not recommend the chronic, long-term use of a spinal support. In almost all patients with some degree of incapacity, we have found that swimming, in a comfortably warm pool, is a useful form of exercise. When the patient cannot swim, exercising in a water environment promotes an equal feeling of well-being, although we have no evidence as yet that either influences bone mass. There is, however, some evidence that exercising on land may prevent subsequent bone loss, if not result in gains in bone mass (Aloia, Cohn, Ostuni, Cane, & Ellis, 1978; Smith, Reddan, & Smith, 1981).

Although such studies conducted with patients who have established disease show some promise, we believe that a more viable use of physical exercise is in prevention of the disorder. Continuity of reasonable exercise patterns from youth is a much more relevant long-term approach to the use of exercise, although undoubtedly we will be faced in the next ten years with an increasing volume of symptomatic patients who require advice about both the potential of exercise programs and their own individual exercise capabilities. At present, regrettably, the advice we as physicians give can only be guarded.

At present, the advice we do offer to such individuals is of a general nature since we have only minimal knowledge of what might be the most appropriate forms of exercise for symptomatic patients, in order to induce increased skeletal mass at sites already prejudiced by excessive bone loss.

SUMMARY

Currently, therefore, although we now have good evidence that bone loss may be prevented or at least retarded when appropriate measures are adopted at an early age, the treatment of those individuals with an already compromised skeleton is more difficult, and the results less satisfactory. In view of the estimated increase in the number of cases of clinical osteoporosis likely to be seen in the United States over the next 20 years, we urgently require a program to increase physician and public awareness of what may become a major public health problem. The unavailability of a good animal model for the disease, and the relative slowness with which results of clinical research can be obtained, indicate that a public awareness program cannot await new scientific information about the causes or treatment of the disease but must start in the near future using the best possible information available to us at present.

6

The Endocrine and Reproductive System of Aged Women

ROBERT B. GREENBLATT,
P. K. NATRAJAN, AND
ANTHONY KARPAS

INTRODUCTION

Life is the continuum of a process known as aging. Anatole France, the French novelist, with great prescience wrote that *"nous étions déjà si vieux quand nous sommes nés"* (we were already old when we are born). Aging begins with one's first breath and surely with the first lusty cry at birth, as if to be born is to start to die. Legend tells of certain heroes upon whom the gods bestowed immortal life, gracing them with that aspect of their own divinity; but the life of man, like that of other animals, moves through the normal span of years between birth and death. Building processes predominate from birth to puberty, then for a varying number of years the building blocks of anabolism and the destructive forces of catabolism reach some sort of equilibrium. When that state of equilibrium is lost, deterioration sets in until one or more bodily systems begin to fail, sometimes with unusual rapidity.

The body machine is designed to self-destruct, and many principles other than anabolic–catabolic ratios are at play to place limitations on one's life span. One of these factors is genetically determined, that is, the capacity for cell renewal. Another concept implicates the body's immune system. The profound deficiency in immunogenesis that occurs with aging could be the consequence of a genetically programmed failure of thymic function. Still another explanation for aging takes into account the interactions between the hypothalmic–pituitary axis and the endocrine system that influences all cellular activity. As an example, ovarian follicles that persist in the postmenopausal ovary fail to respond to rising levels of gonadotropins, resulting in failure of the ovaries to produce estradiol; thus the female climacteric. An understanding of the endocrine and reproductive system in the aged female is central to any study of her physical and mental health.

THE HYPOTHALAMIC–PITUITARY AXIS

Is the integrity of the hypothalamic–pituitary axis intact in the aged woman? Insulin-induced hypoglycemia provokes even a greater growth hormone response in younger women (Roth, Glick, Yalow, & Benson, 1963). The secretion of adrenocorticotropin (ACTH) is also responsive to such a challenge, but to a lesser degree (Blichert-Toft, 1978). Administration of hypothalamic thryotropin releasing factor, TRF, causes a similar response by the pituitary in old and young (Ingbar, 1978). Postmenopausal women maintain very high levels of follicle stimulating hormone (FSH) and luteinizing hormone (LH) for 20 to 30 years before a decline occurs. In the postmenopausal woman in whom high gonadotropins already exist, an injection of 100 μg of the hypothalamic releasing hormone, GnRH, results in an excellent increase in FSH and LH. Prolactin (PRL) secretion by the pituitary is somewhat less than in younger women, but the response to stimulation remains good. One may say then that the axis is not materially impaired in the aged woman, but more data need to be gathered before a definitive statement can be made.

There is, however, a considerable change in cerebral neurohumors; the reservoir of dopamine, norepinephrine, and serotonin in the neurons of the hypothalamus varies according to hormonal status of the woman (Fuxe, 1964). Thus, in the postmenopausal woman an increase in monoamine-oxidase activity coincides with the augmentation of gonadotropins and decline in prolacting secretion: all three related to the estrogen deficiency. The administration of estrogens lowers FSH and LH while increasing PRL levels.

Other disorders of the pituitary, such as acquired hypopituitarism, prolactinoma, and chromophobe adenoma, are observed but seldom in the aged. Acromegaly occasionally blooms in old age, probably having started insidiously several years earlier. The features of the disease are the same as in the younger woman: bossing of the forehead, prognathic chin, large hands and feet, and an increase in size of tongue and internal organs.

THE THYROID GLAND

Investigators have looked for abnormalities in thyroid hormone economy to account for changes in the aging process. An increase in thyroglobulin antibodies is demonstrable in about 20 percent of women by the eighth decade (Evans, Woodrow, McDougall, Chew, & Evans, 1967). Thyroid radioiodine uptake apparently undergoes no marked or significant change with age (Oddie, Myhill, Pirnique, & Fisher, 1968). Large doses of TRF given intramuscularly increase serum thyroid stimulating hormone (TSH) concentration in all women, young and old, but the subsequent rise in serum T_3 concentration lessens with aging (Azizi et al., 1975). The pituitary is the primary sensor of the adequacy of thyroid hormone supplied to the peripheral tissues. Very slight deficiency of thyroid hormone results in increased basal secretion of TSH and response to TRF. In mild hypothyroidism, elevations of serum TSH concentrations may be so slight as to be questionable, but the exaggerated response of serum TSH concentrations to TRF administration readily confirms the diagnosis.

As to thyroid disorders in the aged woman, hyperthyroidism is occasionally encountered. Toxic nodular goiter is relatively more common; less than half over the age of 60 have the typical diffusely enlarged thyroid of Grave's disease. About 20 percent have no palpable thyromegaly and only a small percentage have recognizable ophthalmopathy. Eye signs are usually lacking in the so-called monosystemic, i.e., referrable to the single organ, such as the cardiovascular system. Weight loss, muscle weakness, and wasting are greater than in the younger patient. T_3 thyrotoxicosis is more common in the elderly.

Spontaneous primary hypothyroidism is primarily a disease of the elderly. Presenting signs and symptoms are lethargy, constipation, cold intolerance, loss of mental and auditory acuity, drying of the skin, and to some degree cardiomegaly. Mild hypothyroidism is frequently overlooked in the elderly; T_4 and TSH concentrations are useful in diagnosis. In administration of substitute thyroid therapy, one is admonished to start with small doses (0.25–0.5 mg) of thyroxin because the adrenals, due to myxedematous accumulation, may be underactive. Large initial doses may provoke an adrenal crisis.

The presence of a thyroid nodule in the elderly is less indicative of malignancy than in a younger patient; nonetheless, the possibility of thyroid cancer must be entertained. Undifferentiated carcinoma is almost entirely a disease of those in the sixth decade or older.

THE PARATHYROIDS

Overproduction of parathyroid hormone in the aged woman is frequently unrecognized because of slow progression of symptoms caused by hypercalcemia: anorexia, constipation, nocturia, thirst, and renal lithiasis (in more than half of the cases). Most cases of hyperparathyroidism are uncovered with the widely used chemical screening panel of the automated laboratory (SMA-22). Loss of estrogen effect on decreasing bone resorption allows for slightly higher serum calcium levels that sometimes prove troublesome in differentiating this disorder from true hyperparathyroidism. Although hyperparathyroidism may occur in all age-groups, about 17 percent is found in women over 60 and 0.3 percent in women 80 to 90 years of age. Bone disease, now rarely observed, is seen more frequently in older women. Usually when the disease starts very late, the symptoms are attributed to other pathological conditions such as malignancy or advancing atherosclerosis.

When symptomatic, the disease manifests itself in four organs: kidneys, GI tract, central nervous system, and skeleton. Polyuria, nausea and vomiting, abdominal distention and pain, somnolence, psychosis, lethargy, and coma are prominent features. At times, early signs of bone involvement such as subperiosteal resorption of the middle phalanx may be found (Genant et al., 1973). Fibrocystic disease of bone, epulis, and loss of dura mater of teeth are now rarely encountered. Bone density by photon absorptiometric analysis shows decreased bone density in 75 percent of cases with primary hyperparathyroidism (Pak et al., 1975). Hypoparathyroidism manifested by tetany and/or convulsions is infrequently seen in the elderly unless it follows extensive neck surgery or damage to the parathyroid gland through radiation.

THE ADRENALS

Whether or not adrenal function is impaired with age has been raised because of the importance of the adrenal response as part of the normal defense reaction of the body to life-threatening stimuli. Thus far, no gross disturbance of the regulating mechanism or the rhythmic diurnal variation of cortisol secretion has been demonstrated. The secretion rate of aldosterone is significantly lower, but the significance of this finding is not clear. A rise in adrenal androgens in response to an intravenous infusion of ACTH does not differ between the young and old (Blichert-Toft, Blichert-Toft, & Jenson, 1970), and normal suppressibility follows dexamethasone administration (Friedman, Green, & Sharland, 1969). Risk of exhaustion of adrenocortical reserves in elderly patients when exposed to prolonged strain is not apparent except in those chronically ill or suffering from chronic malnutrition (Cooke, James, Landon, & Wynn, 1964). Under surgical stress, no signs of impaired adrenal reserve capacity have been found with age.

Adrenal diseases in old age are extremely rare. Cortisol-producing adrenal neoplasms and tumors with ectopic ACTH production are on record. Severe hypokalemia and loss of weight rather than obesity may be the presenting signs in Cushing's syndrome. Virilizing adrenal tumors have been encountered. Primary aldosteronism (tumor or hyperplasia) should be suspected in elderly women with hypertension, especially in the presence of hypokalemia, headaches, nocturia, and intermittent attacks of paralysis. The diagnosis is made by the finding of elevated aldosterone levels and low values for plasma renin. Although Addison's disease is rarely diagnosed after the age of 40, one should be on guard for the occasional case. Bronchial carcinoma has been known to metastasize to the adrenal glands, leading to hypoadrenalism. Pheochromocytoma is a well described entity that occurs occasionally in the elderly. The primary source of excessive production of catecholamines to account for the paroxysmal attacks of hypertension may be difficult to locate. Fortunately alpha and beta blocking agents are able to hold such patients in check.

THE ISLETS OF LANGERHANS

Over half of the population at age 70 have abnormal one- or two-hour postprandial glucose values. Although there is a decaying glucose tolerance with age, there is no evidence of a change in tissue sensitivity to insulin with age (Andres & Tobin, 1975). However, if only persons with an elevated fasting plasma or serum glucose value of 140 mg% are diagnosed as diabetic, the incidence decreases considerably. Serious complications, such as retinopathy and nephropathy, are not high among persons with onset of diabetes late in life. The development of cataracts, however, is quite frequent, and symptoms related to neuropathy are often the first evidence of diabetes.

THE OVARY

The senescent ovary is smaller and more fibrotic than in the reproductive years and presents a typical wrinkled, prune-like appearance. In general, microscopic examination reveals a striking diminution of primordial follicles and an increase in amount of connective tissue. At the time of menopause, only a few thousand follicles remain, but these no longer respond to even a tenfold increase in gonadotropin output. The stroma, the source of steroid synthesis in the aging ovary, does not appear to undergo atrophic changes, but may actually increase, resulting in stromal hyperplasia. Thecal interstitial glands are still very common and appear to be well-differentiated, even in ovaries of women many years after the cessation of menses. Activity of the stromal cells may be surmised by the fact that nests of stromal cells may be found in the ovarian mesenchyma that stain for fat with Sudan III and also with special strains for 6-glucose phosphate dehydrogenase, just as do the theca cells of the ripening follicle and the luteinized granulosa and theca lutein cells of the corpus luteum. Between 30 and 40 percent of women over 55 years of age present marked ovarian stromal hyperplasia at autopsy. Its relation with diseases such as endometrial carcinoma, adenomatous hyperplasia, and endometrial polyps is often alluded to in the literature.

ESTROGEN PRODUCTION
IN THE AGED WOMAN

It is well established that the steroid production and secretion of the postmenopausal ovary are altered from those of the reproductive-age years. This alteration is chiefly due to the loss of production of estradiol *de novo* while androgen production continues.

Total urinary estrogens do not differ significantly in the first ten years of postmenopause, but later decrease markedly (Grattarola, Secreto, & Recchione, 1975). The major origin of estrogens in the postmenopause is through the peripheral conversion of androgens. Poortman, Thijssen, and Schwarz (1973) stated: "It is likely that after the menopause all estrogens are derived from peripheral conversion of androgens, without secretion by the ovaries." Ovarian estradiol (E_2) secretion in the menopausal woman is minimal according to the studies of Barlow, Emerson, and Saxena (1969) and Rader, Flickinger, de Villa, Mikuta, and Mikhail (1973). Supporting this, Bulbrook and Greenwood (1957), Procope (1968), and Judd, Lucas, and Yeh (1976) did not find significant alterations of mean E_2 blood levels after gonadectomy in postmenopausal subjects. Sherman, West, and Korenman (1976) demonstrated lower estradiol secretion during the menstrual cycle in the perimenopausal woman, suggesting a decreased capacity of the residual follicles to produce E_2.

In a recent clinical experiment on menopausal and normal women, ovarian, adrenal, and peripheral vein blood were obtained by catheterization, and samples were obtained before and after the intravenous injection of 5000 IU of human chorionic gonadotropin (hCG). Ovarian vein E_2 levels were two to three times lower than in the normal premenopausal woman during the follicular phase (Figure 6.1) (Greenblatt, Colle, & Mahesh, 1976). Injection of hCG did not evoke a significant increase of E_2 production by the menopausal ovary and IV ACTH administration failed to stimulate ovarian or adrenal estradiol (Figure 6.2). The extragonadal conversion of androgens to estrogens is the explanation for the presence of estrogens in the climacteric patient—a level insufficient in most instances to maintain a healthy vaginal mucosa and flora. The prevalent concept that compensatory estrogen production by the adrenal occurs during menopause is not supportable.

ANDROGEN PRODUCTION IN THE AGED FEMALE

The climacteric ovary loses its capability to aromatize sex steroids; the lack of conversion of Δ^4-androstenedione ($\Delta^4 A$) to estrone (E_1), and testosterone (T) to estradiol, results in increased androgen secretion. Judd, Judd, Lucas, and Yeh (1974)

FIGURE 6.1   **Estradiol production in pre- and postmenopausal ovaries.**
In order to determine how the postmenopausal ovary differs
from the ovary of the woman in her reproductive years,
5000 IU of human chorionic gonadotropin (hCG) was administered intravenously and blood collected at 0, 10, 20,
and 30 minutes from a peripheral vein and from the ovarian
and adrenal veins by catheterization. Neither the menopausal
ovary nor the adrenal showed any response by an increase in
estradiol levels, while the ovary in the young woman showed
an excellent response. It would appear from the experiment
that the ovary does not produce *de novo*—the main ovarian
estrogen is estradiol.

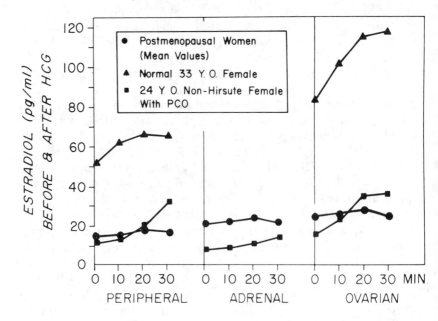

reported the results of ovarian and peripheral vein blood values of
androgens in menopausal women. The mean ovarian T levels were
15-fold higher than in the anticubital vein, and Δ^4A was 4 to 5
times higher. Judd and co-workers concluded that ovarian Δ^4A
and T secretion is greater in postmenopausal than in premenopausal women.

A similar study was performed by Greenblatt et al. (1976)
with ovarian stimulation employing 5000 IU of hCG IV. The
results presented in Table 6.1 indicate that levels of Δ^4A are
much higher in ovarian vein blood (2.3 ± 0.28 ng/ml) in the

FIGURE 6.2   **Effect of ACTH (40 IU) administration on T, Δ^4A and E levels.** In order to prove that the low circulating levels of estradiol in the postmenopausal woman does not come from the ovaries or adrenals but by conversion from androgens produced by the adrenals, 40 IU of ACTH was administered intravenously and blood was obtained at 0, 10, 20, and 30 minutes. There was no increase in estradiol output by either the ovary or adrenal but there was a sharp rise in testosterone and Δ^4-androstenedione levels in the adrenal vein blood.

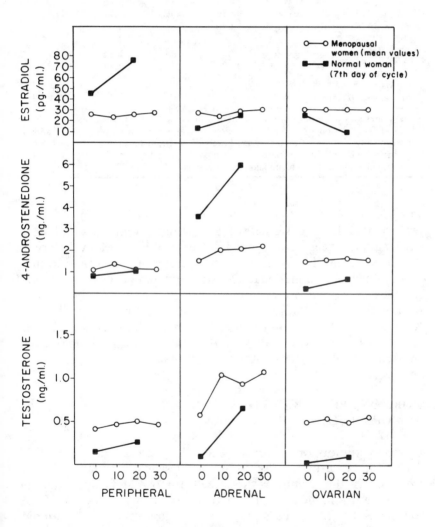

Table 6.1
Serum Delta 4-Androstenedione (ng/ml) Levels in Six
Postmenopausal Women[a]

| | | | | | Δ^4-Androstenedione (ng/ml) | | |
Patient	Age LMP Years		FSH LH mU/ml		Periph.	Adren.	Ovar.
C. F.	52	0.5	53.84	43.11	1.15	1.64	2.33
Z. G.	73	27	32.25	48.76	0.59	1.27	1.73
S. M.	75	15	69.56	38.48	0.93	1.38	1.57
H. L.	58	> 5	93.6	43.2	1.63	2.01	3.22
F. J.	33	4	82.1	38.6	1.14	2.13	2.77
W. T.	60	14	83.11	91.9	1.47	1.87	2.22
Mean values: 6 Postmenopausal Women					1.15±0.17	1.72±0.14	2.3±0.28
Mean values: 10 Normal Adult Females					1.47		1.72

[a]The source of circulating estrone in the postmenopausal woman is believed to derive from the conversion of Δ^4-androstenedione—an androgen produced by the adrenal and probably the stroma of the ovary. Levels of Δ^4-androstenedione was much higher in ovarian and adrenal vein blood of six postmenopausal women than in the peripheral vein blood of both premenopausal and menopausal women.

menopausal woman than in normal women (1.72 ng/ml). Peripheral vein (1.15 ± 0.17 ng/ml) and adrenal vein blood (1.72 ± 0.14 ng/ml) levels are also much lower than in ovarian vein blood. T values are also higher in the menopausal group, and significantly higher than in postmenopausal peripheral and adrenal vein blood samples. Both androstenedione and T rose dramatically in three of the four patients studied 30 minutes after the injection of hCG; the former was much higher than the latter. Greenblatt et al. (1976) concluded that T production by the postmenopausal ovary is twofold higher than in the nonhirsute female.

HORMONE-PRODUCING OVARIAN
TUMORS IN THE AGING WOMAN

Incretory tumors of the ovary occur in postmenopausal ovaries. These tumors usually arise from the mesenchyma and the most frequent is the granulosa-theca cell tumor. Metastatic tumors of the ovary induce stromal activity to steroid production, or the metastatic tumor cells may have hormonal potential. Dermoid tumors, Brenner tumors, and even pseudomucinous cyst adenomas and carcinomas may present with signs of androgen production— either from hormone-producing cells in the neoplasm or, more likely, from stimulation of the contiguous or adjoining stroma. Even in granulosa cell tumors, cells of the tumor may be devoid of lipid-staining granules, but the adjacent stroma frequently shows a lipid deposition resembling the lipoid-laden theca surrounding the growing follicle. Certain ovarian tumors, primary or secondary, may produce other than steroid secretions such as gonadotropins, parathormone, ACTH, and even thyroxine.

Previous literature classified the tumors only according to the clinical hormonal activity (estrogen and/or androgen producing). However, a lack of correlation between clinical expression, laboratory assays, and histology of the tumor (J. M. Morris, 1961) caused confusion among clinicians because of many cases of apparently hormonally bivalent tumors. At the present time, classification of this controversial yet intriguing type of ovarian neoplasm is based on the histology of the cell tumor, independent of the hormonal activity. These functional tumors may have the capacity to produce estrogens, progesterone, androgens, and corticosteroids. Gonadal enlargement is not always present and their occurrence is suspected only because of the presence of an endocrinopathy.

ESTROGEN DEFICIENCY IN THE AGING WOMAN

The consensus has been that vasomotor instability (hot flushes, sweats) and atrophic vaginitis are the only signs and symptoms resulting from estrogen deficiency. Hitherto, mood changes and psychogenic manifestations, so frequently associated with the "change of life," have been regarded as purely coincidental and nonhormone-related. Recent reports by Dennerstein, Laby, Burrows, and Hyman (1978), Moaz and Durst (1979), Lauritzen (1973), and J. W. W. Studd (personal communication, 1982), employing estrogens and a placebo in double-blind studies, have shown that such manifestations as depression, anxiety, and headaches, if not hormone-dependent frequently are hormone-responsive. The implication is that estrogens are psychotonic agents.

Depression

A scientifically based explanation has been offered (Alyward, 1973) in the demonstration that plasma levels of free tryptophan are low in menopausal women with depression, and that estrogens restore these levels. Serotonin is a by-product of tryptophan. Our own studies report Alyward's findings of disturbed tryptophan metabolism (Greenblatt, Nezhat, Roesel, & Natrajan, 1979). We found that the ratio of total to free tryptophan was restored to normal by the administration of estrogens (Figure 6.3).

Experimental studies on mice have shown that brain norepinephrine increases as estrogen decreases following castration, and that T administration on day 1 prevents the normal twelfth-day rise in serotonin (Ladosky & Gaziri, 1979). Fuxe (1964) found that an imbalance in cerebral neurohormones is associated with mood changes such as depression, crying spells, irascibility, nervousness, and change in sexual behavior. Instability of adrenergic and cholinergic cerebral hormones is now believed to result from a deficiency of estrogen. The monoamine-oxidase content of the

FIGURE 6.3   **Metabolism of tryptophan and postmenopausal depression.**
The metabolism of tryptophan (a cerebral neurotransmitter or hormone) is believed disturbed in women with postmenopausal depression. After a six-month trial of estrogens, the ratio of total-to-free tryptophan was restored to the levels seen in nondepressed women.

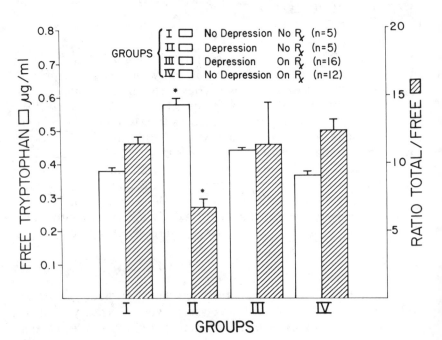

brain matches the prodigious production of gonadotropins by the pituitary in estrogen-deficiency states. To argue that nonpsychotic depression and other mood changes are not hormone-dependent in the menopausal woman is to ignore the role of cerebral hormones (dopamine, norepinephrine, serotonin) in hypothalamic-pituitary physiology. Nonetheless, many excellent students of the menopause believe, as does Utian (1975), that the neurovegetative symptoms such as headaches, fatigue, depressive moods, irritability, loss of libido, and palpitations are most likely part of the psycho-social-cultural phenomena and aging changes that occur in this period of life. Klaiber, Broverman, Vogel, and Kobayashi (1979) have shown that the administration of large estrogen doses reduces monoamine oxidase.

Menopausal Headaches

Many menopausal women with migrainoid headaches relate that during their reproductive years they experienced menstrual headaches that were held in abeyance during pregnancy. Menstrual headache may be delayed through postponement of the menstrual period for 5 or 6 days by means of the intramuscular injection of 10 mg of estradiol valerate one week before the expected onset of the period (Somerville, 1972). The administration of a potent estrogen–progestogen oral contraceptive, started on day 20 of the cycle for 20 or more days, may postpone the headache by delaying menstruation, as has been shown by the delay-of-menses test (Greenblatt & Rose, 1962). Menopausal women with frequent migrainoid headaches often obtain relief for prolonged periods if estrogens can be sustained at high levels. Thus, administration of 1 or 2 pellets of estradiol (preferably with 1 or 2 pellets of testosterone) has proved surprisingly efficacious in a goodly percentage of cases. The headaches often return as the estrogen levels fall after the fifth month. If the headaches experienced by menopausal women are caused by disturbances in the levels of cerebral amines, it is conceivable that hormones may favorably modify their metabolism.

Sexual Dysfunction

Sexual libido is a complex phenomenon that can be studied only in the human. State of health, psychogenic, anatomic, neurologic, and hormonal factors play important roles. Many sex therapists believe that most of the problems of sexual dysfunction are psychogenic, and should be so treated. Sexual dysfunction in the postmenopausal woman may be attributable to dryness of the vagina causing dyspareunia. Estrogens usually are helpful. In women in whom estrogens are not helpful, the addition of androgens to the regimen usually is most rewarding.

Greenblatt, Barfield, Garner, Calk, and Harrod (1950), in a double-blind study of women under treatment for severe hot flushes, noted that the preparation containing a mixture of estrogen and androgens improved libido. Recently, Studd (1979) demonstrated in a double-blind study that estradiol-testosterone pellet implants increased the frequency and intensity of the sexual climax, whereas estradiol pellets and placebos did little to enhance this type of response.

CONCLUSIONS

The only endocrine gland to undergo regressive change with age is the ovary. Accordingly, the age of onset and intensity of symptoms of the estrogen deficiency are not constant because ovarian estrogen production ceases slowly in some women and abruptly in others. Heredity, racial factors, social conditions, parity, and gynecologic and/or general diseases probably are factors in the chronology of menopausal onset. The clinical manifestations of the postmenopausal syndrome, summarized in Table 6.2, can be grouped into three etiological categories: (1) hypothalamic, (2) psychogenic, and (3) metabolic. Many symptoms associated with this period of life may or may not be due to the climacteric. Total awareness of the syndrome permits the physician the orientation in diagnosing the oligosymptomatic forms and lessens the possibility of confusion with other diseases usually present at this age. While the existence of a syndrome caused by the lack or decrease of ovarian function is universally accepted, unanimity does not exist concerning the best way to manage the menopausal patient. Disagreement exists about whom to treat, when therapy should begin, what hormones should be used, and for how long treatment should be extended. Our opinion is that once the signs or symptoms of estrogen deficiency occur, therapy should be instituted and continued for as long a period as possible. Several reports about the association of endometrial carcinoma with estrogen administration are cause for alarm (Smith,

Table 6.2
Etiological Characteristics of the Climacteric[a]

Autonomic N. S.	Psychogenic	Metabolic
Hot flashes	Apprehension	Demineralization
Formication	Depression	Myalgia
Globus hystericus	Insomnia	Skin atrophy
Perspiration	Nervousness	Atrophic vaginitis
Spasms	← Headaches →	Incontinence
Palpitations	← Increase in sexual → responsiveness	Arthritism
G. I. disorders	← Decrease in sexual → responsiveness	Change in lipid metabolism

[a]The conventional view of many physicians limits the symptoms of the climacteric to vasomotor disturbances (hot flushes and sweats) and atrophic vaginitis. More recently an extended view of the menopause takes into consideration autonomic nervous system imbalance, psychogenic disorders, and metabolic disturbances. Only in recent years has demineralization of bone (osteoporosis) in the menopausal woman been linked to estrogen deprivation. Although one cannot be certain to what degree the psychosomatic disorders seen in the menopause are hormone-dependent, symptoms are often hormone-responsive.

Prentice, Thompson, & Herrmann, 1975; Ziel & Finkle, 1975). However, in our personal experience and that of other investigators who have used natural estrogens to induce cyclic withdrawal bleeding at regular intervals with a seven to ten day course of an oral progestogen, the incidence of neoplasia in patients with long-term estrogen therapy has remained minimal (Gambrell, 1978; Greenblatt, Stoddard, & King, 1966). Estrogens may be administered orally, intramuscularly, or by pellet implantation according to the needs and convenience of the patient. The addition of a small amount of an androgen to the estrogenic regimen often enhances the therapeutic effects. An extended view of the menopause permits the inclusion of many symptoms common to the aging woman that may or may not be hormone-dependent but are frequently hormone-responsive.

Hormones will not stay the aging process, will not erase the wrinkled brow, nor lift the sagging breast, but they can help a woman to grow old with grace and dignity. The transition to the climacteric can be eased by the proper administration of hormone-replacement therapy. Treatment should be extended as long as it proves beneficial to the patient's psyche and soma.

PART III
MENTAL HEALTH ISSUES

This section deals with two mental health problems as they are experienced by older women—depression and confusion. In Chapter 7 Holzer, Leaf, and Weissman present data from the 1980 New Haven epidemiologic catchment area survey, which collected data using an instrument that obtained sufficient information for applying the DSM-III diagnostic criteria for depression. Although women had higher rates of depression than men for all age-groups, older women experienced lower rates of depression than younger women. These researchers posited that depression in older women was an extension of the process as it exists in younger women. The issue of treatment was highlighted by the finding that of the 23 older women found to be depressed (1.6% of those 65–74 years of age, and 1.2% of those 75 and older) only three saw a mental health professional for therapy.

Chapter 8 deals with individual therapy and presents the developmental perspective for the treatment of depression in older women, as used by Gutmann and others in the Older Adult Program of Northwestern University Medical School. As an alternative to the "depletion" perspective, which views the older woman as the victim of irreversible losses, the developmental perspective envisions the older woman as the postparental kin-tender in a transition to a new phase of aggressiveness and managerial androgyny. This is a drastic developmental change, and the meanings ascribed to that change are crucial to the healthy emergence of older women's new energies. Gutmann presents the job of the therapist as helping older women clients detach negative meanings from these changes, taking into account the location of change on the internal–external change continuum.

Chapter 9 takes a naturalistic look at 20 years in the lives of three elite old-old women. Wolanin posits that change is the crucial element that threatens these women's ability to maintain contact with reality as these women become increasingly aged and frail. Each of these three women would seem to have successfully traversed the internal changes discussed by Gutmann, and achieved strong, aggressive self-managed lives. However, certain external changes were very powerful, notably closing one's own home and entering a nursing home as a permanent resident. Wolanin describes an episode of confusion in the life of Mrs. H., who experienced this change, and the restoration of her mental clarity following a combination of rehydration, nutritional replacement, and intensive social support. Indeed, Wolanin posits that the ability to handle episodic confusional states depends upon the strength of social support systems in relation to the intensity of the change being experienced.

This section on mental health of older women provides a rather positive perspective. Depression is of low incidence in older women (although higher than in older men) and promises to be treatable from a developmental viewpoint that envisions the older woman as a growing, changing person. Confusion is presented as episodic rather than chronic for old-old women, and episodic confusion is presented as preventable and treatable with strong social support interventions. However, few older women with depression were receiving therapy of any kind, and many women who enter an episode of confusion may not be provided with care that results in regaining mental clarity. Much remains to be done in translating these promises into human care to benefit the older woman experiencing depression and/or confusion.

M. S.

7
Living with Depression

CHARLES E. HOLZER III,
PHILIP J. LEAF, AND
MYRNA M. WEISSMAN

INTRODUCTION

This chapter focuses on aging women. In it, we will make three major points: First, it is important to make a clear distinction between the presence of depressive symptomatology and the occurrence of major depression as a clinical entity. Second, although there is a longstanding belief that depression is particularly prevalent in aging women, recent studies using diagnostic instruments in the community suggest that rates are no higher among elderly than among younger women, and may even decrease with age. Third, studies of the efficacy of treatment for depression suggest that the elderly may be as responsive as younger persons to a variety of standard treatments. Depression, therefore, either in its prevalence or in its treatment responsiveness, should not be accepted as a necessary part of the aging process.

ACKNOWLEDGMENT OF NIMH and NIA. The Epidemiologic Catchment Area Program is a series of five epidemiologic research studies performed by independent research teams in collaboration with staff of the Division of Biometry and Epidemiology of the National Institute of Mental Health. The NIMH Principal Collaborators are Darrel A. Regier, Ben Z. Locke, and William W. Eaton; the NIMH Project Officer is Carl A. Taube. The Principal Investigators and Co-Investigators from the five sites are Yale University—Jerome K. Myers, Myrna M. Weissman, and Gary Tischler; Johns Hopkins University—Morton Kramer, Ernest Gruenberg, and Sam Shapiro; Washington University, St. Louis—Lee N. Robins, John Helzer, and Jack Croghan; Duke University—Dan Blazer and Linda George; University of California, Los Angeles—Richard Hough, Marvin Karno, Javier Escobar, and Audrey Burnam.

The oversampling of elderly respondents in New Haven was made possible through supplementary funding provided by the National Institute on Aging, with Jacob Brody as their representative.

DEPRESSION AMONG AGED WOMEN

There is no doubt that depression is one of the psychiatric conditions affecting aging women. The exact prevalence of depression among elderly women, however, is not well known because of the exclusion of the elderly from many community psychiatric surveys. Furthermore, there have been wide variations in the definition of depression in previous community studies.

Historically, the term depression has been used to identify general states of sadness or dysphoria as well as more restrictively defined disease entities. The variety in the definitions of depression has been reflected in the different studies, resulting in a broad range of estimated prevalence. Most estimates of depression have been based on symptom scales such as those of Zung (1965), Warheit, Holzer, and Schwab (1973), or the Center for Epidemiological Studies Depression scale (Radloff, 1977). When administered in the community these scales reveal levels of symptomatology but do not provide a diagnosis of depression in terms used by most clinicians.

Further, these scales are heavily weighted on physical symptoms that may be produced in the absence of depression by the physical illness so often present in the aged (Blazer & Williams, 1980). Rating scales for use in clinical settings have been developed by Hamilton (1960, 1967), A. J. Beck (1973), and many others. Most of these scales quantify the severity of depressive symptoms without providing a clear guideline for differentiating between the presence and absence of depression as a clinical disorder. Some instruments have the additional requirement that the evaluation be conducted by a clinician, and thus are extremely expensive to use in field surveys. A small number of studies have made use of psychiatrists to conduct direct psychiatric interviews in community settings, but most of these have been limited in sample size and have focused on small communities, limiting generalization from their findings.

As a consequence of the above methodological limitations, there was little firm evidence prior to 1975 about the prevalence of psychiatric disorders such as major depression, even though a number of studies of depressive symptomatology had been conducted.

SEX DIFFERENCES IN DEPRESSION

The increased rate of depression among women of all ages has been thoroughly documented by Weissman and Klerman (1977). In their review they note variability in the assessment of depression, but a nearly universal excess of depression in females as compared to males. Sex ratios for females relative to males ranged from 1.6 to 3.8 in community studies, with the mode being around 2.0. After considering the variety of evidence and alternative explanations for these sex ratios of depression, they concluded that the evidence for an excess of depression in females was real and not an artifact of reporting or help-seeking behavior. Further, they concluded it was unlikely that any one explanation, whether genetic or environmental, would account for the differences found.

AGE DIFFERENCES IN DEPRESSION

Knowledge of the prevalence of depression in the aged is less firm. Conventional wisdom in both psychiatry and gerontology has held that emotional disorder, particularly depression and organic brain diseases, increase greatly among the aged. Butler (1975, p. 893) reported that "Functional disorders—notably depressions and paranoid states—increase steadily with each decade. . . ." This view, however, fails to note the diversity in the literature both in findings and in methodologies used to assess depression. Gurland (1976) provides a review differentiating population studies based mainly on diagnosis from studies based mainly on symptoms. He concludes that "depressive disorders as diagnosed by psychiatrists are most frequent between the ages of 25 and 65" (Gurland, p. 290), while for symptom-based studies "the highest rates of depressive symptoms are found in age groups above 65 years of age" (p. 290). Gurland speculates on whether this difference is a consequence of a psychiatric bias against diagnosing depression among the elderly, or whether some of the symptoms being observed were not due to a psychiatric cause. Blazer and Williams (1980) make the latter point more explicit by examining respondents identified as depressed by a symptom measure, and differentiating the depressed group into primary depression, secondary depression, medically related depression, and dysphoria. The overall prevalence of the depressive state was 14.7 percent of an elderly community sample, while only 1.8 percent had "primary depression" equivalent to the DSM-III operational definition. Thus, measurement procedures may contribute heavily to differences in rates of depression observed in the community.

THE 1975 NEW HAVEN
COMMUNITY SURVEY

A milestone in the development of instruments for diagnostic assessment was the Schedule for Affective Disorders and Schizophrenia (SADS) developed by Spitzer, Endicott and Robins (1978). The SADS provides a structured assessment of symptom content by a clinician with a formal set of diagnostic criteria for establishing a diagnosis. Those criteria, which antedated the current DSM-III criteria, were called the Research Diagnostic Criteria (RDC). Although the SADS was developed primarily for use in clinical settings, Weissman and Myers (1980) saw an opportunity to apply formal diagnostic criteria in a community setting, and therefore used the SADS as part of a follow-up of over 500 respondents in a community survey. In that study they replicated the sex differences for depression in finding that prevalence rates of major or minor depression overall were higher for women than for men, but they also found that the differences became less pronounced in the older age-groups. However, the age differences in rates were less clear, with the peak prevalence of depression for women being found in the 46 to 55 age-group rather than later (Weissman, 1979, p. 195). Rates for men peaked at age 66 to 75 but declined in the 75+ age-group. Although that study had many limitations, particularly being a follow-up of a community rather than the initial sample and having a relatively small sample size ($N = 500$), it broke new ground by being one of the first in this country to attempt psychiatric diagnosis in a community survey.

THE 1980 NEW HAVEN EPIDEMIOLOGIC
CATCHMENT AREA SURVEY

In 1978 the American Psychiatric Association (APA) adopted a revised psychiatric nomenclature that operationalized criteria for psychiatric diagnoses. That document, including the set of definitions it encompasses, is the *Diagnostic and Statistical Manual,* third edition (APA, 1980). Relevant to the present discussion are the DSM-III criteria for Major Depressive Episode (APA, 1980, pp. 213–215), which are summarized in Table 7.1. To meet the criteria, a person must be dysphoric and have symptoms present from at least four different groups for at least two weeks.

Although DSM-III provides criteria, it does not provide a standard interview schedule for assessing the symptoms used in those criteria. The need for such an interview schedule was clear from the work of the President's Commission on Mental Illness, which found very little firm data on the incidence and prevalence of mental illness in the United States. As a result, the National Institute of Mental Health commissioned the development of an instrument that could be used by lay interviewers in community settings to obtain sufficient information for applying the DSM-III diagnostic criteria for a number of disorders. That instrument, developed by Robins, Helzer, Croughan, and Ratcliffe (1981), is called the NIMH Diagnostic Interview Schedule (DIS).

The DIS enabled NIMH to launch a major new program, the Epidemiologic Catchment Area Program (ECA), for ascertaining

TABLE 7.1
Diagnostic Criteria for Major Depressive Episode[a]

A. Dysphoric Mood: depressed, sad, blue, hopeless, low, irritable, prominent, and relatively persistent

B. Symptoms present in four groups for at least two weeks:
Group 1: poor appetite, weight loss, increased appetite, or weight gain
Group 2: insomnia, or hypersomnia
Group 3: psychomotor agitation, or psychomotor retardation
Group 4: loss of interest/pleasure in activities, or decreased sex drive
Group 5: loss of energy, or fatigue
Group 6: feelings of worthlessness, self-reproach, or excessive/inappropriate guilt
Group 7: diminished ability to think/concentrate, e.g., slowed thinking, or indecisiveness
Group 8: thoughts of death, suicidal ideation, wishes to be dead, or suicide attempt

C. Absence of preoccupation with mood–incongruent delusion or hallucination, and absence of bizarre behavior

D. Not superimposed on schizophrenia, schizophreniform disorder or paranoid disorder

E. Not due to organic mental disorder or uncomplicated bereavement

[a]From *Diagnostic and Statistical Manual of Mental Disorders* (APA, 1980).

the incidence and prevalence of psychiatric disorders in the community. The ECA program presently consists of five sites in the United States, each using the DIS to estimate incidence and prevalence of psychiatric disorders in their local mental health catchment areas. Yale was the first of those sites funded by NIMH, with 3000 DIS interviews to be administered in the community. Before the study actually began, additional funding was provided by the National Institute on Aging (NIA) to conduct interviews with 2000 additional persons aged 65 or older. The data being presented here are drawn from the first wave of the Yale ECA project.

Population. The respondents for this survey were selected from the noninstitutional population of 13 towns of the New Haven SMSA. The total population of this area is approximately 420,021, with 262,750 residents between the ages of 18 and 64 years and an additional 51,227 residents aged 65 or older. Less than half a percent of those under age 65 are inmates of institutions, while 1.7 percent of those aged 65 to 74 and 10.7 percent of those aged 75 or more are inmates of institutions and therefore are not included in the present sample, although a separate institutional survey is being conducted as part of the ECA project.

Sample. Two separate but related samples were drawn from this population using a two-stage systematic probability sampling technique. The first sample consisted of approximately 4000 designated respondents aged 18 or older. The second sample, made possible by NIA, consisted of approximately 2776 additional designated respondents aged 65 or more, screened from approximately 12,000 community households. These were designated by first systematically sampling households from utility listings in clusters of eight. Within each cluster the first and fourth household was designated for the community sample. The entire adult population of each house was then listed and a single designated respondent was selected according to a random process described by Kish (1965). The remaining six households of each cluster were designated for the elderly oversample so that only persons aged 65 or greater were listed. One designated elderly respondent was selected using the Kish method. After allowance for vacancies and businesses, and a response rate of approximately 75 percent, interviews were completed with 3058 of the community respondents and 1977 in the elderly oversample.

Interviewing. Interviews were conducted by lay interviewers who had received six days of classroom training with additional practice in the field before being tested for competence with the interview. Close supervision was provided by our field office. The reliability of lay interviewers using the Diagnostic Interview Schedule has been reported by Robins et al. (1981). Interviews were usually conducted in the respondents' homes and took an average of 70 minutes to complete. In some instances the respondent was unable to respond directly to the interview because of a physical or mental handicap or language difficulties. In those instances we attempted to obtain information about the respondent from another member of the household, or a relative, by administering a proxy interview. Approximately 150 proxy interviews were completed during the course of the study.

Instrumentation. The interview schedule consisted mainly of the NIMH Diagnostic Interview Schedule with questions added to obtain demographics, mental health utilization, and related variables. The MiniMental Status Exam (MMSE) of Folstein, Folstein, and McHugh (1975) was also included.

The Yale interview uses Version 2 of the Diagnostic Interview Schedule (Robins et al., 1981). Sections covering 13 major categories of disorder were included. These are listed in Table 7.2.

The section covering major depressive episode is directly parallel to the DSM-III criteria presented in Table 7.1. This section begins with a question on dysphoria, feeling sad or blue, followed implicitly by a series of probes that determine whether the re-

TABLE 7.2
DSM-III Diagnoses from DIS Included in
New Haven Survey

---

1. Alcohol dependence
2. Anorexia nervosa
3. Antisocial personality
4. Drug abuse or dependence
5. Dysthymia
6. Major depression
7. Manic disorder (bipolar)
8. Obsessive compulsive
9. Panic
10. Agoraphobia
11. Simple phobia
12. Schizophrenia
13. Somatization
14. Cognitive impairment, based on MiniMental Status Exam

---

spondent went to a doctor because of the dysphoria, whether he/ she took medication for it, or whether it interfered with his/her life. Then the respondent is asked whether he/she has ever had any of a series of 16 depressive symptoms that correspond to the 8 symptom groups of DSM-III. An attempt is made to determine whether these symptoms cluster with the dysphoria, if indeed dysphoria is reported, and whether the time the most symptoms occurred also had an equivalent to dysphoria. That period in either instance is defined as the "worst period." The first and last experience of such a symptom cluster is determined, as well as the number of episodes experienced. For the "worst period" only, the respondent is asked to recall whether each of the 16 symptoms was present. The presence of dysphoria and at least one symptom in four DSM-III symptom groups is sufficient to meet the basic criteria.

Additional criteria are present in DSM-III requiring that the symptomatology not be the result of uncomplicated bereavement, manic disorder, schizophrenia, or organic brain disease. The issue of bereavement is tapped by two questions asking whether the depressive episode occurred "just after someone close to you died," and whether it occurred at any other time. Exclusions for other disorders are based on the results of other diagnostic sections of the DIS. They are not being applied formally here but their effect would be small.

RESULTS

Characteristics of the Sample

Table 7.3 provides a description of two demographic characteristics of the community sample and elderly oversample, age and gender. As can be seen from the age distribution, there are a large number of elderly of both sexes in the study, particularly when the elderly from both samples are combined. Large samples are required for the study of psychiatric disorders because of the small proportion of the population affected by any specific one of them.

TABLE 7.3
Age and Gender Characteristics of Sample

	Males		Females	
Age of Respondent	Number	Percent	Number	Percent
18–29	345	16.8	462	15.6
30–44	373	18.1	477	16.1
45–64	337	16.4	452	15.3
65–74	691	33.6	918	31.0
75+	311	15.1	652	22.0
Total	2057	100.0	2961	100.0

Prevalence of Depression
by Age and Sex

The first major issue in the present analysis is the prevalence of depression as distributed by age and sex. Table 7.4 presents prevalence rates for the six-month period preceding the date of interview. Two relationships dominate this table. First, the prevalence of depression is higher for women of all ages. This relationship is emphasized by the female/male sex ratio within each category, which ranges from 1.3 for the middle-age category to a maximum of 4.4 for the 30 to 44 age category. The sex ratio is intermediate for the two oldest age categories. This sex ratio is consistent with most of the recent literature.

The second trend in this table is that depression, as assessed in this study, is highest in the youngest two age categories and generally declines with age. Although the prevalence of depression for elderly women is higher than for elderly men, it is lower than for the younger men and much lower than for younger women.

Before proceeding, one possible explanation for this result should be ruled out. That is the possibility that the exclusion of bereavement is greatly reducing the rates for the elderly where loss of close friends is more common than for younger age-groups. That is in fact the case for the older respondents, particularly females. With bereavement included, the prevalence for females in the age 65 to 74 category jumps from 1.6 percent to 2.7 percent. Within the 75 and up age-group the prevalence increases from 1.2 percent to 2.0 percent. Nevertheless, as Table 7.4 shows, the pat-

TABLE 7.4
Sex- and Age-Specific Prevalence of Depression Bereavement for the Six Months Preceding the Interview[a]

	Total Number	Depressed		Bereaved		Total	
		N	%	N	%	N	%
Males							
18–29	345	16	4.6	0	0.0	16	4.6
30–44	373	7	1.9	0	0.0	7	1.9
45–64	337	6	1.8	1	0.3	7	2.1
65–74	691	4	0.6	4	0.6	8	1.2
75+	311	2	0.6	1	0.3	3	1.0
Females							
18–29	462	33	7.1	1	0.2	34	7.4
30–44	477	40	8.4	2	0.4	42	8.8
45–64	452	11	2.4	3	0.7	14.	3.1
65–74	918	15	1.6	10	1.1	25	2.7
75+	652	8	1.2	5	0.8	13	2.0
Sex Ratio							
18–29	1.4		1.5		–		1.6
30–44	1.3		4.4		–		4.6
45–64	1.3		1.3		–		1.5
65–74	1.3		2.7		–		2.3
75+	2.1		2.0		–		2.0

[a]These figures are based on the unweighted counts from the combined Wave I community and elderly oversample.

tern of general decrease with age persists as do the sex ratios for each of the age categories.

This finding is consistent with previous diagnostic studies in the New Haven area (Weissman & Myers, 1980) but is inconsistent with much conventional wisdom about the elderly and research findings based primarily on symptom measures. These previous studies, however, may have overestimated the prevalence of depression among the elderly because of the presence of physical symptoms that mimic depression and because of the use of assessments that fail to differentiate between dysphoric states associated with the situation of the elderly and the more narrowly defined clinical disorders of major depression.

Risk Factors

A second major issue is the set of conditions that are associated with depression as risk factors. A proper ascertainment of risk factors would require a study of incidence rather than prevalence, because one cannot be certain that any particular factor is a cause of the depression rather than being the result of a current or previous disorder.

Table 7.5 presents the prevalence of depression for women aged 65 or more by marital status and living arrangement. Higher prevalence of depression is found for the separated or divorced than for other groups. The lowest prevalence for depression proper is reported for the widowed, a rate of 1.3 percent, but that rate is somewhat confounded by the exclusion rule for bereavement. All but one of the 15 elderly women reporting bereavement fall within the widowed category. It may be that some of these additional respondents represent a severity of disorder beyond the uncomplicated bereavement excluded from depression by DSM-III. Were that true for all 14 bereaved widows, the rate of depression for that category would increase to 2.8 percent, making it the marital status with the highest prevalence of depression. The issue of exclusions is a complicated one calling for judgments of causality

TABLE 7.5
Six-Month Prevalence of Depression for Women Aged 65 or Over
by Marital Status and Living Arrangements

	Total Number	Depressed		Bereaved		Total	
		N	%	N	%	N	%
Marital Status							
Married	413	7	1.7	1	0.2	8	1.9
Widowed	940	12	1.3	14	1.5	26	2.8
Sep. or div.	93	2	2.2	0	0.0	2	2.2
Single-never married	123	2	1.6	0	0.0	2	1.6
Living Arrangements							
Living alone	796	11	1.4	8	1.0	19	2.4
Lives with spouse	337	4	1.2	1	0.3	5	1.5
Lives with child or parent	151	4	2.6	1	0.7	5	3.3
Other	286	4	1.4	5	1.8	9	3.2

that are well beyond the limitations of the DIS as administered by lay interviewers.

Table 7.5 also presents the association between living arrangements and depression for these elderly females. The most common arrangement was for the respondent to live alone, accounting for 51 percent of the respondents. Twenty-one percent of the respondents lived with their spouses and 10 percent lived with either a child of theirs or, in only six cases, a parent. The remaining 18 percent lived with someone else of undefined relationship. As expected, the lowest prevalence of depression was found for those living with spouse. Surprisingly, the highest prevalence, 2.6 percent, was found for those living with a child or parent. While this result may be due to the small sample size, it is interesting that the respondents expected to receive high social support would be that depressed. One might wonder what other processes affect this relationship.

Low social status is also considered a risk factor for depression. Table 7.6 presents the prevalence of depression by education and income. The highest prevalence of depression is found within the lowest education category, corresponding to elementary education only. Interestingly, the second highest prevalence is found in the category that includes those who attended college for at least a year. The relationship between depression and the respondent's reported income is only suggestive, with slighly lower prevalence of depression in the high income category, but when bereavement is included, that category has the highest rates.

Additional risk factors such as race and employment were considered, with no differences being discovered. This may be a result of the relatively small sample size, but it may also result from the general character of these aging women as survivors.

Age at Onset

In the previous section we have examined the relationship between various factors associated with depression, but have neglected the possibility that the depression being reported is a process of long standing that antedates the current situation. To examine that question we have looked at the reported age the respondent first experienced a depressive episode. Because this is based on recall, it cannot be taken uncritically, but it should be indicative of the presence or absence of a history of depression.

TABLE 7.6
Six-Month Prevalence of Depression for Women Aged 65 and
Over by Income and Education

	Total Number	Depressed		Bereaved		Total	
		N	%	N	%	N	%
Income							
0–4999	399	8	2.0	1	0.3	9	2.3
5000–9999	404	8	2.2	3	0.7	12	3.0
10,000 +	412	6	1.5	8	1.9	14	3.4
Education							
0–6	175	6	3.4	3	1.7	9	5.1
7–11	711	6	0.8	7	1.0	13	1.8
12	348	5	1.4	1	0.3	6	1.7
13+	336	6	1.8	4	1.2	10	3.0

We have data on 23 women meeting the criteria for depression. Of these, only 5 (24%) reported onset after the age of 65. One respondent could not identify an age of onset, 9 (41%) had onset between ages of 45 and 64, and the remaining 8 (36%) reported onset before the age of 45. For bereavement the picture was somewhat different. Of the 14 respondents reporting bereavement, 10 (71%) reported having first experienced a depressive episode since the age of 65. Thus, bereavement is more likely than major depression to have its origin in the period after age 65.

The above findings, although tentative, indicate the need to deal with the origins of depression in terms of incidence rather than the prevalence rates available. The simple association of depression with the various risk variables is not enough to establish a causative relationship. As the present study proceeds, reinterview data will be available on these same respondents, which will permit us to examine these etiological issues in a more rigorous fashion. For the present, however, we must conclude that there is no evidence for a special set of mechanisms being operative among elderly female respondents. The relatively low prevalence of depression coupled with the lack of etiological leads, suggests that depression in the elderly is very much an extension of the depressive process active with younger females. Many of those who have experienced depression at a younger age continue to experience depression later in life, while a relatively small number of women experience depression for the first time after the age of 65. Bereavement, on the other hand, appears to be somewhat more common, particularly as a new disorder, although it appears that at least some of the bereavement being reported is of prolonged duration and thus may go beyond the uncomplicated bereavement that DSM-III excludes from depression.

Symptom Profile

One additional question about the character of depression is raised by the literature. There exists the possibility that the phenomenon of depression as experienced by elderly women is somewhat different from depression as experienced by younger women. In order to examine that question, all women ever having experienced depression were divided into three groups based on their current ages and the age at which they experienced their worst episode of depression. This identified 160 women younger than 65 who by definition had experienced their worst period of depression (obviously) prior to the age of 65. A second group of 21 women were over the age of 65, but reported a worst episode prior to the age of 65. Finally, 17 women aged 65 or older reported worst episodes of depression after reaching the age of 65. This procedure of reporting depression based on the "worst period" is made necessary by the lifetime focus of the DIS and its reliance on "worst period" for making a diagnosis.

Having distinguished between episodes of depression experienced before or after the age of 65 by the elderly cohort, and the depression experienced before the age 65 by the younger cohort, it is possible to ask whether there is anything unique about the depressive symptomatology experienced by elderly women. Table 7.7 presents the 16 depressive symptoms combined into 8 symptom groups used as criteria in the DSM-III. One must have 4 of these symptom groups to meet DSM-III criteria.

Examination of Table 7.7 reveals a general similarity between the symptom profiles reported by each group. The major differences found were that the elderly woman experiencing a worst episode after the age of 65 were more likely to be positive on group 3, "slow-restless." That group includes reporting feeling tired out all the time, moving more slowly than normal, or having to be moving all the time. This excess may result from the physical limitations of being older. Two symptom clusters were markedly lower than expected among the elderly, the appetite cluster

TABLE 7.7
Symptom Groups for Depressed Respondents
by Age and Period of Worst Episode

DSM-III Symptom Group	Age <65 Episode <65 N = 160 (%)	Age 65+ Episode <65 N = 21 (%)	Age 65+ Episode 65+ N = 17 (%)
Appetite	78	76	53
Sleep	88	81	88
Slow-restless	53	48	76
Lost interest in sex	29	19	0
Tired	75	71	76
Worthless	68	52	65
Thinking	84	71	82
Thoughts of death	76	67	65

and the loss of interest in sex. These may be low because they are attributed by respondents to the aging process and thus are not considered as part of depression. Overall, however, the symptom patterns are highly similar, suggesting that depression for these elderly females is very much the same process as depression among younger women.

THE ISSUE OF TREATMENT

The final issue in this chapter is the extent to which treatment reduces the impact of depression on elderly women. When the 23 depressed women were asked about their use of mental health services, only 3 (13%) reported having seen a mental health specialist such as a psychiatrist, psychologist, or social worker within the six months prior to interview. An additional 6 (26%) respondents had seen their medical doctor about mental health problems, making a total of 9 (39%) of the depressed elderly women seeking some kind of treatment. In fact, only 12 (52%) of these depressed women reported ever having received mental health care for any reason. Similarly, only 5 (33%) of the bereaved women had seen their medical doctors about their mental health, and none of them had been to a mental health specialist during the previous six months.

This low level of utilization, even for those women with major depression, suggests that the respondents or their physicians, or both, may consider their depression to be unavoidable and not treatable, or their depression may not be recognized at all. The lack of treatment for these depressed women represents the self-fulfilling prophecy embodied in the title of this chapter, because recent studies suggest that the elderly respond well to various treatments for depression. Therefore the elderly should not have to live with even the levels of depression reported here.

8

Developmental Perspectives on the Diagnosis and Treatment of Psychiatric Illness in the Older Woman

DAVID L. GUTMANN

ORIGINS OF STRESSFUL CHANGE

This chapter will present, briefly, some conceptions regarding the sources and consequences of stressful change, particularly as it affects the diagnosis and psychiatric treatment of middle-aged and older women. These conceptions have been generated by the faculty and students of the Older Adult Program (OAP) of Northwestern University Medical School, in the course of bringing developmental conceptions to bear on clinical work with this population. Thus, in the interest of developing more hopeful and more realistic alternatives to the "depletion" perspectives that now dominate geropsychiatry, the OAP personnel have been identifying developmental contributions to the pathogenic stressors of later life.

Stress may reach pathological levels when the individual is involved in transitions—developmental or otherwise—that lead to unfamiliar stimulation (pleasurable as well as unpleasurable) of the sort that demands unfamiliar responses—those that are outside of the individual's practiced, familiar affective and behavioral repertoire. Developmental processes provoke transitions; particularly at their outset, they bring the individual into contact with stress-inducing stimulation of the sort defined above: in the outer world, and within the precincts of the self. As such, developmental processes constitute one source of stressful change, and of psychopathology. Accordingly, the clinical importance of autonomous developmental processes has to do with the fact that they induce stressful change as the necessary price of growth and new structures.

In order better to understand the developmental contributions to late-onset psychopathology, we will first consider the more general relationship between stressful change and psychopathology, as well as the ways whereby the *meanings* associated with such transitions—developmental or otherwise—can render change more or less pathogenic. We begin by considering, in greater depth, the variable of change.

Drastic change has various sources, ranging from internal to external, as well as various outcomes, ranging from the largely reversible to the fixed and irreversible. At the "internal" end of the *internal–external* change continuum, we group endogenous or eruptive forms of change, brought on by the emergence of innate developmental potentials, toward new appetites, new learning, new capacities, and new forms of social participation. Given sponsoring environmental conditions, such changes are stimulated by internal "clocks" or by specific "chemico-social" signals for which the individual has a heightened, phase-specific sensitivity. Thus, a 16-year-old boy would be sensitive to sexual overtures from females that he would not have noticed—or would have noticed in a different way—at the age of 10. The potentials released by innate change are dynamic and proactive: they compel the individual to seek out new settings, in which the new potentials can be exercised, disciplined, and trained, to become executive capacities of the individual self, as well as resources for some larger social unit.

Midway along the *internal–external* continuum, we group *reciprocal* sources of change. Here individual change and transition results from the intersection and collaboration between hitherto dormant self-potentials and the agents that facilitate or welcome them. As examples, we think of individuals who are forced by necessity to exercise hidden talents they had long put aside, and in consequence discover some latent gifts of courage, leadership, or physical dexterity. We also think of individuals liberated by changing imposed circumstances (such as retirement) to seek out new settings, those where they can train and exercise talents that had never developed beyond the eruptive, unformed state.

Finally, at the most *external* pole of the change continuum, we group changes imposed from the outside. These can have significant consequences for the individual even though they come about without any collaboration between the psychological system of the individual and the change-inducing agents. This category of change includes all imposed and usually irreversible losses, whether these originate in the individual's body, his or her circle of kin and intimates, workplace, or larger social world. Here, we refer to bodily losses resulting from infectious or degenerative processes; of losses of loved persons through death, desertion, social upheaval; of losses of employment or of economic opportunity brought on by wars, famines, or depressions. Finally, at the macro-social level we refer to those losses of national leaders and prestige that may cause a crisis of spiritual morale in the individual citizen.

THE INTERSECTION OF CHANGE AND MEANING

Even those changes that entail irreversible loss do not necessarily lead to psychological disasters; whatever the source of the transition, the personal consequences of any change are mediated by the *meanings* that the individual identifies with these dislocations. Thus, endogenous changes, which normally initiate new appetites and new strengths, may acquire malignant meanings, particularly if the emerging potentials stimulate dangerous unconscious fantasies, as well as unacceptable excitements, pleasures, and triumphs. Thus, while most adolescents bloom with new sexual vigor, a significant minority are frightened by their new sensual endowment: for them, these appetites may provoke unconscious incestuous fantasies, centered on tabooed parental figures. Conversely, for some individuals, drastic imposed losses may have beneficial rather than damaging consequences in certain life domains: the loss of physical vigor can provide passive men with a needed excuse to get out of the "rat race" with honor, perhaps to pursue less renumerative but more personally satisfying careers. In some cases, the loss of a person—even one who is truly loved—may have the ultimate effect of liberating the survivor to pursue an expanded but hitherto unavailable lifestyle.

Thus, just as change can be initiated from inner or outer sources, the meaning of a change can also stem from various sources: it can derive from cultural consensus; it can derive from unconscious, idiosyncratic associations; and finally, it can derive from the individual's subjective apperception or translation of the normal cultural meanings associated with a particular change.

In sum, to understand the psychological impact of any significant change, we must locate it on an *internal-external* change continuum, taking into account the nature of the change, the source of the change, and the source and nature of the cultural and/or personal meanings that attach to the change.

In those cases where change has had a noxious effect that calls for intervention, the usefulness of any remedy will also be affected by the same factors that mediate the impact of change. Thus, when there is clear congruence between imposed, irreversible losses and negative meanings, such cases call for remedies against the (usually) reversible symptoms—for example, the *pains* of loss—rather than the pathogenic losses themselves. On the other hand, those that stem from eruptive, endogenous change call for remedies against the reversible aspects of the pathogenic conditions, rather than against the symptoms alone. In these instances, we consider the distance between the actual changes, as these are normally understood, and the idiosyncratic meanings that the patient has assigned to them. Has a potential growth process been misperceived, turned into a pathogen, by virtue of the idiosyncratic meanings that the patient has mistakenly attached to it?

In those cases where losses are externally imposed and (usually) irreversible, our remedies partake of the same external nature: we use chemotherapy to relieve symptoms, and we try to replace the lost object by altering the patient's social conditions. But when the shock is internal, when potential growth is experienced *as though* it portended catastrophic and irremediable loss, then our therapy deals with the inner symbolic world rather than the external object world. More precisely, we seek in such cases to correct the incongruity between the eruptive event and the frightening meanings that have clustered around it and falsified its true nature. At the internal, symbolic level of events, therapists need not be coerced by the patient's catastrophic illusions; they can alter destructive (but reversible) process through corrective interpretations, so as to replace inappropriately bad meanings with benign and realistic meanings that are more congruent with the emerging developmental potentials.

CHANGE AND MEANING
IN CURRENT GEROPSYCHIATRY

Thus, we see that both change and meaning can derive from a wide spectrum of sources and that they can interact in myriad ways, where each combination can have a distinct consequence for pathology and treatment. However, when geropsychologists and geropsychiatrists consider the plight of the older female patient, they almost invariably restrict their attention to one limited combination of change and meaning to explain the pathology and to define the remedy. According to modern geropsychiatry, the cause of disease is invariably an external, imposed and irreversible loss, whether of health, beauty, fertility, or "love object," and no distance or tension is perceived between such losses and their painful meanings. The patient is truly a victim of arbitrary deprivations, and she has no reason to believe otherwise. Therapy consists of providing sympathy and support, while attempting to allay the pain of inevitable loss, usually through chemotherapy.

Thus, when change is presumed to entail irreversible loss and ascribed meanings are entirely consistent with the traumatic changes, then meaning has been ruled out as an independent and reversible contributor to the pathology, or as a pivot for potential therapeutic intervention. Also disregarded is the possibility that eruptive changes, presaging growth rather than decline, may provide a basis, even in women's middle years, for late-onset pathology. But this neglect of developmental possibilities in pathology flies in the face of much research evidence, from this and other quite different cultures, all of which make the point that the post-parental years are not necessarily a time of irretrievable loss. Rather, this may be a time when change is provoked by the endogenous emergence of new potentials; linked to positive meanings, these can lead to the revitalization of the older woman. But modified by negative meanings, these same changes can author drastic psychopathology.

We will briefly review some of the more dramatic evidence for developmental change, particularly that coming from cultures more patriarchal than our own, those where women's lives are particularly constrained by social customs. Thus, this author and other ethnographic investigators have, working independently of each other, amassed evidence of a very robust and quite profound developmental onset in postparental humans, one that is most clearly observed among older women.

THE VITAL OLDER WOMAN:
CROSS-CULTURAL FINDINGS

During the preparental and parental years, younger women concede to their male protectors, whether blood kin or husbands, their own aggressive potentials. They look to their husbands for protection, expecting them to defend the perimeter of the domestic zone against those human enemies and animal predators that would menace them and their children; and they look to their husbands to either supply nutriment and shelter for their families or to defend the space in which these physical supplies are secured. In short, younger women look to their husbands for the provision of physical security, and they also expect them to be exporters of aggression: They rely on male partners to move aggressive forces—including their own—out of the domestic zone, where they could put children at risk, and to deploy such energies in a useful way against enemies and physical nature on the frontiers of the community. However, once their children are grown and able to supply their own physical and emotional security, once their children are no longer vulnerable to the parents' —and particularly the mother's—aggression, older women reclaim for themselves the aggressive potentials that they once sent out of the house with their husbands. They emerge in a confidently assertive form, often as the ruling matriarch of the extended family and its physical environs. Across the planet, wherever we find extended families to be the major corporate bodies within organized societies, they are very often ruled—*de jure* or *de facto* —by older women. These tough old wives generally oversee and command—often in concert with their oldest sons—a host of daughters-in-law (the "servants" that their sons have brought home in marriage).

In effect then, the older woman—*precisely because she is older, and past the childrearing stage*—has a particularly vital role to play, in crucial aspects of social and individual maintenance. Her aggression, which will no longer damage her children or drive away the male provider, now fits her for an expanded administrative role, that of *kin-tender*. Her care is no longer devoted to the children of her body, but to the more impersonal management of a larger and more enduring social unit—the extended family. The large and intimidating family to which she was brought as a young bride now becomes her assured domain. It is an object for her in the fullest psychological sense, and her continuity as a person is intimately identified with the continuity of the family that she monitors, controls, and represents.

In sum, if psychological development entails the predictable emergence of structured, reliable capacities that enhance the well-being of the individual, as well as the maturation of other individuals, then older women clearly undergo a profound developmental change in later life, and show aggressive and managerial powers that were only latent in their makeup before this post-parental advance. In effect, they become androgynous, sexually bimodal, a mixture, as many observers have put it, of mother and father.

THE VITAL OLDER FEMALE: PRIMATE FINDINGS

Recent studies of aging among subhuman primates provide inter-species evidence for the clear developmental shift in the post-parental female that was first developed through intercultural comparisons. Bear in mind that certain crucial similarities across the primates allow us to make what are more than accidental inter-species comparisons. Most significantly, human and subhuman primates have in common the long dependency and vulnerability of infancy and childhood. In both the ape and human cases, the primate infant may have—as we begin to discover—some precocious communicative and social skills, but it is almost completely lacking in the skills that ensure physical security: It can hardly move in any coherent fashion, it certainly cannot remove itself from danger, and it can barely secure its own milk. Among the lower primates the infant has, at best, the capacity to cling, during the first year of life, to its mother's fur. Of necessity then, adult primates—whether human or otherwise—have in common an intense concern with parenting, and this concern is particularly manifested in the behavior of reproductive females. Thus, like the majority of younger human mothers, the mother ape is devoted almost exclusively to the care of the latest infant, the one still clinging to her fur. She is at the same time relatively inoffensive in her dealings with other adults, and largely relies on dominant males, rather than on her own teeth and limbs, for the physical protection of herself and her current infant. During the period of intense parenting, she allies herself with physically dominant males and trades sexual access for their protection. However, in the postparental years, a striking change occurs, one which parallels our cross-cultural observations among humans. Hrdy (1981), who conducted field studies of the Langur and Macaque monkeys, has noted that the ways in which older monkeys support younger animals seems to vary with the sex of the animal and the situation of the group. Males generally bow out leaving older females to intervene actively in the fate of their descendants. In effect, female primates have two roles in regard to procreation. They provide physical as well as emotional security—though, consistent with the exclusivity of these roles, they play them out sequentially, rather than concurrently. Hrdy reports that when a troop of Langurs is threatened by dogs or humans, or by encroachments upon its territory by other Langurs, it is typically the adult male *or the oldest females* who leave the rest of the troop and slap at the offenders.

Interestingly, the primate evidence shows that older female apes devote their care and protection, as "mothers" and as "fathers," not to the youngest babies, but to those who have separated from the mother's fur, the "toddlers" who are now at risk not only from external predators, but also from the same adult males who protected them, as infants, in exchange for their mother's sexual favors. Thus, by becoming in effect both mother and father, the postreproductive grandmother supplies, in an interim and transitional fashion, the maternal love and the paternal protection that is no longer available to the child once it has physically separated from the biological mother. By becoming sexually bimodal, the postreproductive female provides a transitional but vital form of parenting, comprising both male and female modes, that guarantees successful outcomes of the crucial and dangerous passage from physical union with the mother to full separation and autonomy.[1]

[1] In this regard, there are striking parallels between the human and the primate data: thus, like subhuman females, human grandmothers often take over the care of those grandchildren who have begun to remove themselves from the orbit of the mother's immediate concern. This is particularly true in those devastated social enclaves where human affairs degrade toward anarchy. In these deculturated settings, the mothers are preoccupied with securing protection for themselves and for their latest infant from some physically strong though often unreliable and even assaultive male. It is the combative, kin-tending grandmother who emotionally nurtures and even physically protects the older, separating child who has become the rival rather than the protégé of the mother's male consort.

Clearly then, postreproductive female primates take up the defender's role that is usually reserved for young and vigorous males. The breeding mothers are almost exclusively providers of emotional security; but like adult males, the postreproductive female moves at times of danger, not to the protected center of the troop, but to its outer defense line. There they take up the "warrior's" role that is, for good evolutionary reasons, off limits to the younger females. In sum, the older postparental women openly reveal the aggressive propensities that would have put their children at risk but that are vital to their expanded role as *kin-tenders*, as administrators of the extended family settings in which parenting goes forward. The late-blooming aggression that would unfit them to be mothers does fit them ideally to administer and protect, not only their grandchildren, but also the breeding mothers in their nutrient enterprise.

Thus, when the primate female, human or subhuman, exits from the active maternal role, she does not end her life cycle, but instead begins a new and potentially more aggressive phase of existence, endowed with a vitality that was much less available during the parenting years (when she was physically more vigorous, but psychologically more inhibited).

DEVELOPMENT, PATHOLOGY AND TREATMENT IN THE OLDER FEMALE

But the eruptive, developmental energies that are released in women by the ending of the "emergency" phase of parenthood can provide the major fuel for later life pathology, as well as further growth and adaptation. These powerful energies can become "untracked" from growth to find covert and unacknowledged expression in wrenching symptoms, instead of significant social roles. This "developmental" pathology comes about—as in adolescence—when the older woman has irrational but compelling reasons to fear her own emerging energies. That is, for idiosyncratic reasons having to do with her personal history, her socialization, or her particular life circumstances, such energies have acquired disastrous meanings for her and have come to imply destruction rather than growth.

A common outcome for such women is to develop, often for the first time, the classic symptoms of an agitated and reactive depression. These symptoms serve to deny the reality of inner change by presenting the patient as a victim (albeit of her own self-inflicted pain) rather than as a potential aggressor. Moreover, since depression is most commonly interpreted as a reaction to external loss, the symptom serves to shift the seeming locus of change away from the inner world to the outer world. Our tentative formulation is that many of these "developmental" casualties may be protecting not only themselves, but also their vulnerable middle-age husbands. By becoming sick and damaged, the wife allows him to externalize his own sense of depletion and keeps him in a strong and protective "masculine" role. Thus, through her depression the mid-life patient is frequently saying to her husband, to her therapist, to herself: "Do not see me as someone who is revealing a destructive nature; rather, see me as the innocent victim of an imposed and unkind fate." In effect, the depression does represent a reaction to loss; but these losses have less to do with external deprivations and more to do with the losses of self-esteem and self-continuity that are provoked internally, by the emergence of an alien entity: the frightening aggressive potentials newly discovered within the self.

Far too many practitioners collaborate with this defensive maneuver, and tacitly concede that the patient's troubles do indeed have external causation. In these instances, there is, in effect, a convergence of defenses between the patient and the practitioner. The patient wants to be seen as externally deprived rather than internally threatened (or threatening); and given the equation in conventional geropsychiatry between loss and depression, the therapist is prone to agree with the patient and to treat her disease as a reaction to harsh external circumstances. In collusion with the patient, the therapist is likely to concentrate on the palliative treatment of symptoms, while ignoring the reversible structure of the disease itself—the tension between potentially positive inner changes and the destructive meanings that are unconsciously and unreasonably associated with such changes. Thus, by ignoring the developmental and unconscious sources of change, the therapist gives up his or her most potent therapeutic leverage over reversible sources of pathology in exchange for a less effective and less dynamic role as drug pusher, shock administrator, and hand-holder.

The hidden threats and possibilities in the female unconscious at mid-life can be made manifest by techniques and instruments that provide the patient with the opportunity to externalize the unconscious urgings—and the fears around these—so as to make them available for analysis and correction. Methods include the sponsorship of transference reactions; the analysis of dreams and early memories; and the analysis of the imagery generated by projective tests, such as the thematic apperception test (TAT) and the Rorschach. For example, consider the Rorschach protocol by a married woman in her mid-50s, who comes to outpatient psychotherapy for the first time in a state of great agitation, complaining of anxiety and depressed mood. She seemed so desperate and needy that her novice therapist considered refusing the case, on the grounds that this patient would be "too draining." Not unlike some experienced therapists, the intern had been taken in by her patient's self-presentation as an empty, incapacitated woman.

However, the diagnostic tests revealed a different picture. Thus, the first response to the Rorschach was of two stags in the mountains, "guarding their territory." Her second response featured two bulls in battle: They have collided and have locked horns so that blood gushes from their open wounds. Her fourth response depicts a "large scary monster that could attack you." Her sixth response proposed an eagle in flight, while her seventh response, an association to a typically "phallic" card area, summarizes the major issues: "It looks like an explosion of something—a coming up to creation. It looks like a butterfly, a beautiful butterfly, but like it broke loose. It's coming out of its cocoon—a beautiful butterfly has emerged . . . out of eruption comes a work of nature. Looks like it would be all rainbow colors, like Niagara Falls. Out of eruption comes a spray of multicolors."

Clearly, this is not the imagery of a depressed woman. This woman is both terrified and fascinated by the aggressive "masculine" strivings that threaten to break through her defenses into consciousness. In her mind, aggressive, "masculine" vitality has acquired catastrophic *meaning*: It connotes murderous struggle (the bloodied, fighting bulls) perhaps involving her husband (the two stags guarding their territory). Thus, her emergent masculine persona has the meaning of and is experienced as an alien monster that attacks her out of the dark wood. However, there is also pleasurable excitement and hope: Out of the volcanic eruption a beautiful butterfly is being born. Clearly, the patient attaches both positive and negative meanings to her crescent energies; and it is the job of the therapist to help her detach the negative meanings, so that she can experience her own vitality in more appropriately positive ways. Thus, her last Rorschach response predicted the course of treatment: Over some months, the patient has come to accept, live out, and even enjoy her no longer hidden wishes, and the depressive symptoms are subsiding. The fearsome volcano is delivering up a butterfly; and this transformation reflects not a change in the energies themselves, but in the meanings that surround them.

Finally, we are not Pollyannas; we do not deny that external loss can be a major factor in many cases of female mid-life depression. However, the case reviewed above is not atypical, and we do argue that therapists should learn to recognize the signature of true developmental transition in mid-life—however masked it may be by catastrophic meanings—as well as the more disastrous, irreversible transitions that currently claim our exclusive attention.

9
The Aging Woman and Confusion

MARY OPAL WOLANIN

Age does not tell us about the differences between older women. We must look at other variables—particularly health. Health at 65, and at 80, and at 90 all have different expectations, and one could not expect the same quality of health at each decade. Socioeconomic status can vary from the poverty stricken, of whom a fair percentage are elderly women, to some of the wealthiest people in this country, who are elderly widows of the very rich. And there are many levels between.

Marital status is another variable, ranging from the married for a half century to the more recently married; and the long widowed to the newly widowed, many of whom are new widows at 80 years of age. There are also the divorced, and the never-married. For the first time in history we have a group of career women who are single, who are retired after autonomous independent lives, and who have their own retirement income based on their earnings instead of those of their husbands or fathers. Social support also will vary widely: there is the woman who has complete confidence that those who love her will always be at her side, in contrast to women who have no real friends or confidantes. Another variable is ability to recall, which studies tell us should be excellent for details that have significance, but which could also fail (Botwinick & Storandt, 1980; Ridley, Bachrach, & Dawson, 1979). All of these variables require a grid with so many possibilities for permutations that we must admit that aging women cannot be discussed as a homogeneous whole—as if at 65 years old women were cut with a life-sized cookie cutter and reshaped into an "aging woman."

I have had the good fortune to know three women who are now 90 or over. I have known them well for 20 years and observed them during the time in which they went from young-old to what could be considered an old-old plus. This is a longitudinal study with a small N, but I did not know at the beginning that I, let alone my three 90-year-olds, would be here 20 years later. So my sample is made of a special group of women who have made it—have come to their ninetieth birthdays in a magnificent way—two of them in possession of the creative and problem-solving ability they have always had. The third has had increasing memory loss since her eighty-seventh birthday. Without her social graces, which are perfect, she could not have lived alone and driven her car until she was 90. She has season tickets for the football games as she has had for 50 years.

To a world that somehow expects that we will be senile if given time, I offer this record. Two were married in their 30s, one lived in a happy marriage for 52 years and the other for over 40 years. The latter one has three children. Both are widows now. The third never married, but she has told me of two great affairs—one of which continues today. The gentleman friend sends valentines, but his frailty prevents his visiting. In fact, it was his inability to visit that coincided with her beginning loss of memory in her eighty-seventh year.

All have splendid health. Of the 20 years I am recording, there has been one hospitalization—for five days. The other two women seldom see a doctor, and to the best of my knowledge they do not take any prescribed medications. The one who was ill, Mrs. H., admitted herself to a nursing home when she found her strength unable to cope with keeping a home, putting fitted sheets over recalcitrant mattress corners, and managing her investments. She put all her property in a trust but kept a bank account, writes her own checks, and balances her own checkbook. Miss T. has never been in a hospital in her life. All three women had very good educations for a generation that has an average educational attainment at sixth grade level.

Miss T. has a Ph.D. from a great university abroad. Mrs. H. has a degree with a major in business from N.Y.U.—unheard of for women in her generation—and Mrs. S. came to this country from Europe at age 16, learned the language, earned her living, and graduated from a School of Nursing in 1916 when she was 27 years of age. She was one of the first industrial nurses in the United States. All have managed their own business affairs. Miss T.

has stock in 35 companies—she loves to read the annual reports and collect dividends. She has never sold a stock, only purchased. Mrs. H. put her affairs in a trust, and Mrs. S. handles her own income.

Each woman has lived in the same home for at least 15 of the past 20 years and the move was made of their own choice. They chose the residence, and it was filled with their possessions—some of which came from their parents as heirlooms. All are involved with community and national affairs. Mrs. S. will discuss the editorial page of the morning paper with you. Mrs. H. is sure that Reaganomics will ruin her. Miss T. uses her morning paper for a TV guide. She now lets her bills lie unopened, and she forgot to pay her income tax this year. When her driver's license expired this May she panicked. She had forgotten what you do to renew it. That was when her family came from another community and closed her house and took her to a nursing home.

All had parents who lived to see them grown to adulthood and established. Each woman had a sense of independence that has been kept throughout her life. Each one looks back on a well-spent life. Miss T. tried to find a single word to describe her life and always still comes out with "sweet."

This has been a great story up to now, but in the past few years sensoriperceptual losses have intervened. Each woman is having increased deafness. Mrs. H. and Mrs. S. have visual problems and find reading quite difficult. Each has used problem solving to maintain contact with the daily newspaper. Miss T. does not wear glasses. She is the only one who has driven her car during the past ten years. Mrs. H. tells me never to give up my driver's license.

I wanted to begin this chapter on a positive note and hope to have made my case that aging does not mean senility. These remarkable women show what happens when people maintain good health and good lives until 90.

On this evidence, then, we cannot say that age alone is responsible for the confusional states that we see in some older women. The following variables seem important in sustaining these women: good health, love and social supports, adequate income, good education, and continuing challenge to their minds with creativity, problem solving, and interest in the world about them. They had good parenting and parents—and they all believed in themselves. They had no sudden changes during the 20 years except Mrs. H.'s widowhood, which was a turning point for her. It is these variables that I would watch as predictors of possible confusional states in older women.

My working hypothesis is that change, rapid change in any area, leads to confusional states: physiological shifts such as in hydration, drugs added or withdrawn, anemia, or any condition that reduces the oxygenation of the brain or changes the glucose available for metabolism. There can be sudden changes in location —geography, which can be as limited as a move into three rooms in the next block from a large home of many years, or a major move across a continent with a change in climate, humidity, and seasons, and mountains where a beach was before. Or it may be bereavement in which one is suddenly alone—very alone after years of companionship. My first question is always "What change has occurred in this person's life?" These may be major changes or smaller changes, as in level of ability to know the world through hearing or seeing. I have an equation that expresses this:

$$\frac{\text{Change}}{\text{Social (family) support system}} = \text{Ability to maintain contact with reality}$$

Small change and a large support system will result in no confusional state of consequence. Let me give you an example with one of my 90-year-olds. Mrs. H. surveyed her situation—her aloneness and inability to manage her home and business affairs, her almost total lack of friends, and no family who could be her support. She admitted herself to a nursing home, and her trust officer arranged to sell her household furnishings, her last responsibility. When they were sold she had no link to her life history except me—and I had not realized that I was to be that link. She became depressed and stopped eating and, worse, stopped drinking fluids. The nurses were very impressed the day she came out into the nurses station and when asked where she was going in her nightgown, announced she was going to pick blueberries in the hills. No one ever picked blueberries in Tucson, let alone in February, which it was. They called me, and after assessing the situation I decided she must have constant care and rehydrating. We hired sitters, who gave her human care, touched her gently, talked with her and read the headlines. Most important of all, the slow job of rehydration and nutrition replacement was begun. She improved at once. I came each day and still see her each week unless I am away. She has my fall schedule and knows where I am at all times. I was her family, her social support system, and when this was increased by three very caring young women, her confusional state cleared as her physical and social situation changed.

At any age one can have reversible confusional states (Wolanin & Phillips, 1981), and at any age recognition of the change from the usual or normal can lead to intervention that can be restorative. This leads to the crucial point in this topic—the aging woman and confusional states. While confusion can occur at any point in a life cycle, the events of the aging woman's life seem to put her at great risk. There is the socioeconomic situation, which for many elderly woman is a step just above if not below the poverty level. The death of her husband often leaves an older woman facing difficult financial affairs for the first time in her life. Households headed by elderly women have a much lower income than households headed by men. And with reduced socioeconomic resources, there is danger of nutritional loss and a diminishing of health care. The changes come rapidly—bereavement, decision making, health status losses due to stress and aging, and often depression. Most can problem solve with support (Denney, 1980), but for many there may be little or no support.

Relocation often forces change even when only from one place in a community to another—from the home of many years' residence to a small apartment. Or it can mean traumatic relocation such as follows a fractured hip, a condition found in one in three older women who live to 90 (Wolanin & Holloway, 1980). Unless adequate social support systems are functioning, the fractured hip may be the big change that will lead to a life of dependence instead of the independent living enjoyed up to that point.

Although Medicare and Medicaid are supposed to cushion the blows of medical expense, only 38 percent of most expense is covered. For the woman with limited financial resources, trying to balance food and medical bills results in losses either way. Without adequate support she may well choose the dignity of paying her bills and eat an iron-poor diet. Confusional states can arise from an anemia that can result in hypoxia. There are still marginal vitamin deficiency states in this country: among the aged, these include vitamin B_{12} deficiency, or pernicious anemia and lack of folic acid. The worst case of pellegra I ever saw was a well-to-do widow who was too lonely and depressed to eat anything that contained the needed vitamin B.

Communication problems result in a false impression of confusional states. Communication must be practiced. It is a learned art and becomes rusty with lack of use, just like piano playing skills. Many aged women literally have no one to talk with. Listening to television and radio is not communicating. The repartee needed in a two-way conversation may be lost (Meyerson, 1976). Ward found that the never-married aged were least likely to counteract their social isolation with community involvement. They are more likely to live alone or with an unrelated person (Ward, 1979). For the single person, poor health and low income lessened the ability to cope (Ward, 1979).

The new widow or the widow from a childless marriage is often one who has been socially isolated, especially if the deceased spouse had a long terminal illness. Such women do not seek community support and may be referred to as socially regressed (Johnson & Catalano, 1981; Smyer, 1980). They lose their communication skills, giving the effect of being confused.

Finally there are the irreversible confusional states associated with senile dementia, either Alzheimer's type or multi-infarct dementia. These may be critical in aging women, depending on the availability of support systems. For the elderly woman who has ample family and social support, the disease may progress into the final stages before institutionalization is needed. Some families prefer to maintain the aged relative in their homes until death. The basis is the family tie, the strength of affectional bonds developed throughout life. When these are absent, even if the family relationship is close, the confusional states can result in either a severe burden on the family—usually a daughter (Archbold, 1980)—or there can be a breakdown of the family with abuse and neglect (Phillips, 1980). Few aged husbands can manage the care of the aging woman with progressive degenerative dementia.

In short, I leave you with the equation that I introduced earlier:

$$\frac{\text{Change}}{\text{Social (family) support system}} = \text{Ability to maintain contact with reality}$$

Even major life changes, if buffered by the existence of an effective social support system, will not diminish an old person's ability to maintain contact with reality and to avoid a confusional state.

PART IV
SOCIAL ISSUES

Women have long been recognized as the guardians of social relations, both within the family and, often, between the family and society. Few health practitioners could now deny that social factors are directly implicated in the etiology, treatment, and management of illness. It is therefore peculiarly appropriate to include, in a book on the mental and physical health of elderly women, some social conditions that affect their lives in old age, and by implication their well-being at all levels. Kin-keeping, dealing with the losses of loved ones, and the quadruple jeopardy of racism, ageism, sexism, and poverty are the issues presented in this section. In each of these chapters, it seems that there are more questions raised than answers provided. More research, especially longitudinal studies, are clearly needed.

The kin-keeping role was found by Hagestad and others to be uniquely that of women in both vertical and lateral family lineages. The implications of this female role on men when mid-life and later-life divorce occurs is discussed. The characteristic themes of attempts at intergenerational influence are presented for the alpha, omega, and mid-generational women. One comes away from the Hagestad paper impressed with the potential strengths of vertical and lateral family ties, and the central role of middle-aged and older women.

Burnside next presents a distillation of selected literature and illustrative cases regarding three of the social losses often experienced by older women—of spouses, children, and pets. The loss of spouse is uniquely different for aged women and aged men. Aged men will have ample opportunity to remarry: aged women only rarely have such an opportunity. Thus grief, often prolonged grief, following widowhood can be expected by most aged women. She notes the common experience of hallucinations about the spouse as comforting to the recently bereaved widow. Burnside concludes by presenting some guidelines for the clinician drawn from the literature and her own experiences.

The third chapter, by Jackson, calls for the development of an ethnogerontology. Problems in operationalizing minority status and poverty status are explored, in the absence of longitudinal studies of these and other distinctive subcultures. The absence of mortality data by socioeconomic status for aged, black women makes it difficult to evaluate or assess the outcomes of triple or quadruple jeopardy. Both theoretical and empirical deficits leave this important area, from a social-policy viewpoint, full of ambiguities and unanswered question.

M. S.

10
Older Women in Intergenerational Relations

GUNHILD O. HAGESTAD

INTRODUCTION

Earlier in this book Dr. Riley discusses women in patterns of societal generations—what we now commonly call cohorts. My focus is on other kinds of generations—those found in family lineages.

We now define generation in a system of ranked descent, or what I like to refer to as *vertical linkages.* Intergenerational relations in the family can be visualized as a set of interlocking, vertical ties that weave together interdependent relationships and interconnected lives. The key linkage in such vertical connections is the parent–child pair. My topic in this chapter is older women in intergenerational relations. Rather than defining "older" by using chronological age, I have chosen to define it in terms of dimension of family time, namely generational processes. My discussion will focus on women who are members of their family's two oldest generations. For some families, that means they have one generation below them; for others, there may be four. In earlier writing, (Hagestad, 1982) I have called the oldest position in a generational structure the *omega.* Individuals in this position are parents, but not children. At the opposite end of the structure are the *alphas.* These family members are children, but not parents. Between these two extremes are individuals who occupy both the role of parent and the role of child. Such individuals are "generational bridges" (Hill, Foote, Aldous, Carlson, & MacDonald, 1970) who connect the young and the old. Using this framework, this chapter concentrates on omega women and their daughters. Throughout my discussion, I argue that it is essential to see such intergenerational pairs in a wider generational context, because their resources, strengths, and strains reflect and are shaped by those of other generations in the family. The need to consider family relationships within a wider generational structure has become increasingly clear as a result of recent demographic change in our society. Let me briefly outline some key aspects of such change.

THE CHANGING DEMOGRAPHY OF INTERGENERATIONAL RELATIONS

Until quite recently in American society, couples considered themselves fortunate if their wedding party included their parents. Today, many weddings include grandparents, and some even have great-grandparents. This contrast is one example of how demographic change has altered the nature of family life in our society. Two aspects of such change are of particular interest here: the unprecedented duration of parent–child ties and the rise of multigenerational families. Among individuals born around the turn of the century, a substantial number lost their parents before reaching adulthood. Uhlenberg (1980) estimates that in the 1900 birth cohort, one of four experienced the death of at least one parent before reaching the age of 15. The corresponding figure for children born in the 1970s is one of 200. In today's society, parents and children expect to spend several decades of shared lives after the children are adults and likely to be parents themselves. Four-generation families are now common (Shanas, 1980); five or six generations in the same family are not unheard of.

The new duration of parent–child relationships and the increasing number of multigenerational families stem from two sets of demographic changes: increased general life expectancy and altered rhythms of family formation. American women now live close to eight decades, but have their children earlier in life than did women in previous historical times. Thus, we have witnessed an "acceleration of generational wheels."

MEN AND WOMEN IN VERTICAL TIES

Women outlive men by nearly eight years. In addition, they typically marry men who are older than they. As a result, mothers and daughters have a more durable, long-term relationship than any other parent–child pair. Winsborough (1980) suggests that when women born in 1930 reach the age of 60, more than one-fourth will still have their mothers living. He further predicts that among women born in 1970, nearly 42 percent will still have their mothers at age 60. These trends mean that more women than men are grandparents of adult grandchildren and more women live to know their great- and even great-great-grandchildren than do men. Thus, younger generations more often have contact with old women than old men in their families, and the oldest family member known to children as they are growing up is likely to be a woman.

Another consequence of differences in mortality between men and women is that most older men are married; most older women are widowed. In 1979, 67 percent of all men over the age of 75 were living with a wife. Only 21 percent of women in the same age category were living with a husband (Uhlenberg & Myers, 1981). That means that men retain a significant *horizontal* generational relationship till the end of their lives, whereas women do not. These differences lead to contrasts in need for support in the face of failing health. Most older men are cared for by their wives; most older women turn to children for help.

Given contrasts in life situations of older men and women, it is reasonable to conclude that women are more involved and invested in vertical family relationships than are men. It is often pointed out that this difference can be observed very early in life.

From a variety of theoretical perspectives, it is argued that women's involvements in the family are both qualitatively and quantitatively different from those of men. In discussions of adult role patterns, women are not only found to spend more time in family roles, they also appear more emotionally invested in them. The Michigan studies of mental health in America (Gurin, Veroff, & Field, 1960) have found women's "ups and downs" related to family happenings, while those for men tend to be connected with the sphere of work. Studies of the life span and its markers suggest that women's turning points are more likely to be related to family changes than is the case for men (Neugarten, 1968; Siegler & George, in press). The stronger family orientation of women has been linked to early socialization and differential personality development in boys and girls. A number of authors have argued that girls grow up with a strong orientation toward interconnections in the interpersonal realm (Brock, von der Lippe, & Block, 1973; Chodorow, 1978; Gilligan, 1982; Hess, 1979). Boys have a stronger focus on active mastery of the world around them.

In research on socialization, it has been found that family obligations and preparation for family roles are stressed more in the upbringing of girls than is the case for boys, and girls understand kinship concepts earlier than boys (Jordan, 1980). Therefore, men and women enter adolescence and young adulthood with quite different self-definitions and role orientations (Block et al., 1973). Women, much more than men, have been groomed to be kin-keepers and "ministers of the interior," that is, focused on the inner familial world and its workings, a difference that lasts a lifetime.

It has also been argued that there is a difference between men and women in their orientations to peers and nonpeers. Specifically, it is suggested that age demarcations are more significant in structuring men's relationships than is the case for women (e.g., Kogan, 1979; Liljestrom, 1971).

In the family, striking differences have been found between men's and women's orientation toward vertical bonds, that is, relations across generational lines. Women's strong early investment in parenthood reflects lifelong differences between the sexes. Men concentrate on relationships with peers and members of their own generation more than women do.

These brief remarks have argued that women and men have differential involvement in vertical family ties. Women not only spend more time in them, they also tend to invest more heavily in such bonds. Thus, they have more "on the line" than do men and are more apt to experience intense rewards as well as risks and problems from such relationships. As Gilligan (1982) puts it: "Women, therefore, are ideally situated to observe the potential in human connection both for care and for oppression" (p. 168).

I now turn to some examples of how older women's involvement in intergenerational relations spells strength and satisfaction, as well as vulnerability and stress. My discussion will concentrate on three aspects of multigenerational living: contact and kinkeeping, intergenerational continuity and conflict, and patterns of interdependence and support. Research illustrations include work by colleagues, as well as two studies in which I have been involved: one focused on patterns of influence in three-generation families and one dealt with divorce in middle age.

In the late 1970s, I was part of a team that studied members of three generations in 148 Chicago area families. From each family, we conducted separate interviews with one young adult grandchild, both the middle-aged mother and father, and one aged grandparent. The basic research design was a dyadic one. Across inter-generational pairs, we asked both members to discuss each other and their relationship. We therefore had reciprocal data, reflecting the two individuals' views of their relationship. The only exception was that the grandparents were not asked to discuss their child-in-law.

During the academic year 1979–1980, M. Smyer and I conducted a study of middle-aged divorce in a metropolitan area (Hagestad, Smyer, & Stierman, 1984). Working from court records, we contacted and interviewed 93 men and women who had been divorced for about one year. The respondents had a mean age of 50. Prior to the divorce, they had been married an average of 25 years. All of them had children, the majority of them young adults. Sixty percent of the respondents also had at least one living parent, ranging in age from the early 60s to the upper 80s. The in-depth interviews concentrated on the divorce process, but obtained considerable information about relationships with the other two generations: maturing children and aging parents.

OLDER WOMEN IN INTERGENERATIONAL RELATIONS

Kinkeeping

Work on kinship patterns has repeatedly demonstrated that contact and exchanges between generations to a large extent are facilitated and carried out by women. In a recent Canadian study (Rosenthal, 1981) nearly 500 individuals over the age of 40 were asked: "Is there currently any one person among you and your family who, in your opinion, works harder than others at keeping the family in touch with one another?" Three-fourths of the respondents named a woman. "Keeping the family in touch" means organizing get-togethers, as well as maintaining contact through letters and phone calls. In their classic study of working class families in East London, Young and Wilmott (1962) suggested that kin ties represented the equivalent of a trade union, organized for and by women. These authors described "Mum" as the hub of family solidarity and cohesion: "The siblings see a good deal of each other because they all see a good deal of Mum" (pp. 57–58). Similarly, Berardo (1967) looked at the rate of interaction with relatives following the death of parents and concluded that:

The role of the father apparently has little import with regard to the maintenance of extended family relations. The interaction level of subjects with a surviving father was almost as low as when both parents were deceased. (p. 553)

In the study of three-generation families in Chicago, we found the same pattern; women bring families together. They organize the get-togethers, remember the birthdays, write the Christmas cards—not only to their own family, but often to their husbands' kin as well. At least in the United States, research has found that wives are often the main link to their husbands' families, as well as to their own relatives (Adams, 1968; Bahr, 1976; Berardo, 1967; Leichter & Mitchell, 1973; Reiss, 1962). In the study of mid-life divorce (Hagestad et al., 1984) many of the men expressed concern about the viability of family bonds. About a third of them said that neither they nor their children ever had strong ties to the paternal grandparents. It is quite possible, judging from other research, that these men had felt closer to their wives' family than to their own. A divorce is likely to sever some valued family bonds for men, and leave them a bit at a loss without a kinkeeper and mediator. One man angrily exclaimed: "Just at the time when I was ready to be with my family, I found that I didn't have one!" On the other hand, early training and years of mothering appeared to have given the women an unshakable faith in the strength of their family ties—a faith that nothing could threaten such ties. Their interviews seemed to carry the message "Of course the children will still have a family—I *am* family!"

Women also observe family relationships more closely and are more likely to register changes in the ways members relate than are men (Hagestad et al., 1984; Wilen, 1979). In the Chicago study, we found that the middle-generation women kept close track of two other generations, their parents or parents-in-law and their children. Indeed, they seemed to have assumed a role of "family monitors." This emphasis on internal family dynamics and the role as "ministers of the interior" also emerged for the two older generations of women in the Chicago study of three-generation families. A major emphasis in this research was patterns of socialization and influence across the generations. It also explored sources of conflict and strain in intergenerational relationships.

Socialization, Continuity, and Conflict

In my view, there are three key aspects of intergenerational socialization. First, there is an ongoing process of negotiating expectations regarding family relationships. Second, family members help one another face and understand a changing world. Third, there is the creation of family continuity.

Several authors have argued that demographic and cultural changes have produced intergenerational roles and relationships that are not clearly defined or structured by societal norms (e.g., Hess & Waring, 1978). People in such relationships have to negotiate a common base for relating through the course of their interaction. Thus, in this view, the process of socialization does not involve the *transmission* of expectations, but the *creation* of them (Bengtson & Black, 1973).

Family members also use one another as resources in dealing with the world *outside* the family. This function of family socialization was the major topic of classic social science discussion. The emphasis was on how parents prepare children for life as adults in society. Increasingly, we have recognized that in a social context characterized by high rates of change, such preparation cannot be done "once and for all," because people become old in a world quite different from that in which they spent their childhood. In the family, the young often serve as "cohort bridges" to older members, by mediating, interpreting, and making human sense of technological and cultural range. A current example from American middle-class families would be young children teaching their parents and grandparents how to use home computers.

A third type of socialization process involves a search for intergenerational continuity. Families work to maintain a sense of communality and similarity—a set of "family ways" or "family themes" that transcends generational boundaries and endures generational turnover. In my view, this process is one of intergenerational transmission from old to young, because it is a question of what is to be passed on to future generations. The more I study families, the more impressed I become by the amount of effort they expend on maintaining a sense of continuity, and by the variability in what they choose as the core of such continuity.

Moreover, men and women differ in where they concentrate efforts to create and maintain continuity.

In exploring the Chicago data, I studied the extent to which the middle generation aimed influence attempts at the young and old. Overall, the middle-aged attempted more influence in relationships with the young. However, about 30 percent reported roughly equal number of influence attempts to old and young and 10 percent said they sent more "up" than "down." Cases in which more influence was aimed at the aging parent than the young adult child most commonly were in families where a widowed grandmother was interviewed. When we examined how the middle-aged respondents discussed attempts on behalf of others to influence *them*, nearly one-half reported equal numbers of such attempts from the child and the parent. Only about 15 percent said the child made more efforts to influence them than did the parent. Thus, a reasonable conclusion seems to be that parents never give up trying!

The one area of influence that cut across all the relationships examined in the study was *health*. Family members in all three generations reported that they struggled to keep the others healthy by trying to get them to watch their diets, stop smoking, see the doctor, and take their medicines. Beyong that, we found considerable variation by generation and gender.

Fathers and grandfathers tended to concentrate influence in areas outside the family domain: work, education, money, the management of time, and social issues. Women in the two older generations concentrated more on interpersonal issues of concern to the family: how to relate, dating, the relative importance of family and friends. Such division between male and female areas of influence was particularly strong in the grandparent generation. Internal family affairs seemed to be defined as women's issues. Some grandfathers expressed that quite correctly in their interviews, flatly declaring interpersonal family issues as "none of their business."

Differences between men and women, particularly grandmothers and grandfathers, also emerged when we asked about "difficult topics" in the intergenerational pairs. The nature of such troublespots showed differences by sex of individuals involved. When grandfathers were discussed, views on social issues were by far the most commonly mentioned. Race relations, social policy, and sex roles were current issues that came up frequently. Between middle generation fathers and the grandchild generation, the most commonly mentioned difficult subjects were related to work, money, or education.

In discussions of grandmothers and mothers, the clear trouble-spots were topics dealing with interpersonal issues, particularly in the family realm. The most frequent mention of such touchy subjects was found among mothers discussing grandmothers. Apparently, two kinkeepers did not always see eye to eye. In their reports, grandmothers, like the other family members, most frequently mentioned interpersonal, family issues as creating difficulties between them and younger generations. These findings are remarkably similar to a recent study of German families (Lehr, 1982). In this research, intergenerational disagreements and arguments among men focused on non-family spheres. Among women, conflict occurred over how to relate in the family.

Some close qualitative analyses of the Chicago data provided further insights into the relative silences of issues *within* the family and relations with the world *outside* the family to men and women in intergenerational relations.

We identified the families that had all-male or all-female lineage connections. The all-male lineage subgroup had a paternal grandfather, a father, and a grandson interviewed. There were 10 such families. The all-female lineage subgroup had a maternal grandmother, a mother, and a granddaughter interviewed. Twenty-four families fell in this pattern. In these 34 families, we again focused on "the straight line" and did not read the middle-generation parents who did not have their own parents interviewed. In close reading of entire family sets of interview protocols, we have concentrated on identifying *themes* (Troll & Bengtson, 1979). In order to be counted as a theme, the same issue had to be brought up by at least two of the three people and indirectly involve all three family members.

There were some striking differences in what men and women paid attention to and talked about in their relationships across generations. For men, themes fell into domains of instrumental concerns (work, education, and money) and social issues in society at large. For women, they were typically focused on interpersonal relations, mostly within the family.

The Chicago data suggest that men and women in the older generations concentrate on different aspects of intergenerational continuity, in ways that are quite similar to Parsons and Bales' (1955) distinction between "instrumental" and "emotional-expressive" leadership. Grandfathers and fathers emphasize

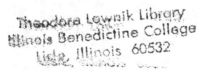

relationships with the wider society through work, education, and finances. Women as grandmothers and mothers concentrate their efforts on relationships *within* the family. At times, there appears to be some conflict between two generations of kinkeepers over how things should go in the family. For both kinds of issues—how to relate to a changing society and how to manage internal affairs, there is a process of mutual influence and negotiations across generations. However, women seem to have more negotiation, that is, influence flowing up *and* down generational lines in their attempts to find a common base for relating. The "hub" of such negotiation is the woman in the middle generation.

This study points to the importance of the mother–daughter link in the maintenance of family cohesion and continuity. Because of their long lives, women spend decades of life when they are both mothers and daughters. Relationships "up" to the mother and "down" to the daughter go through multiple seasons of rewards and stresses, vulnerabilities and strengths. Recent discussions of intergenerational support has pointed to the pivotal role of middle generation daughters in providing necessary help to aged parents.

Patterns of Support and Interdependence

A sizable research literature has explored patterns of exchange across the generations. Repeatedly, it has been shown that even though modern society does not have an extended family structure, there is an impressive exchange of gifts and services between older people and their children. However, little work has explored the flow of support and concern "up" and "down" generational lines within families.

In some early research I was struck by questionnaire responses from nearly 800 undergraduate students who were asked about their relationships with their parents. The majority of both male and female students said their mother was more likely than their father to discuss personal problems and worries with them. Recent work on primary relationships in later adulthood has found that women, significantly more than men, use children as confidants (e.g., Babchuk, 1978). Our study of divorce in middle age (Hagestad et al., 1984) found similar trends.

Two findings stood out from Babchuk's study. First, during the divorce process, women utilized their "vertical connections" to parents and children more than men did. Women more frequently turned to the two other generations to discuss marital problems and to seek emotional and material support. Second, when family supports were relied on during the divorce process, children were both turned to more and seen as more helpful than parents, especially by women. Two-thirds of the women, compared to one-fourth of them, said they had discussed their marital problems with their children. When the respondents were asked to identify the person who was the most helpful during the worst part of the divorce process, nearly one-fourth of the women named a child. Five percent of the men did so. Our data suggest that women, more than men, approached children as adult equals, to whom they could turn for advice and support. Parents were also turned to by a number of our respondents. Three-fourths of the women and half of the men who had surviving parents said they had discussed marital problems with them. However, only *one* respondent in the sample mentioned a parent as most helpful during the crisis of marital break-up. The tendency for these middle-aged individuals, particularly women, to rely more on help from grown children than from aging parents made me curious about whether this in part reflected negative attitudes toward divorce on behalf of the parent. In some recent pilot interviews with middle-aged women we asked them: "If you had a personal problem or worry, would you discuss it with your parent or your (oldest) child, do you think?" More than half of them (54%) said the child, less than a fourth (21%) said the parent.

So far, I have concentrated on members of the middle generation as recipients of support from parents and children. Much recent discussion has focused on the middle-aged as *providers* of support and concern.

Again, the pivotal role of women has been highlighted. A number of authors have talked about "women in the middle" (Brody, 1982), also called "the sandwich generation" (Schwartz, 1979) and "the caught generation" (Neugarten, 1979). Brody points out that they are in middle age, a middle generation, and find themselves in the middle of competing demands on their time and energy.

It has been well documented that most elderly prefer independent living. However, many of them face a time in advanced old age when they require steady care. It is estimated that 80 percent of such care is provided by family, usually daughters (Troll, Miller, & Atchley, 1979). When an old person moves in with a middle-aged child, it is typically a mother moving in with a daughter. It is estimated that of elderly parents living in such arrangements, eight out of ten are mothers, and two-thirds of them are living with a daughter (Troll et al., 1979). A study at the University of Michigan found that among middle-aged children housing elderly parents in need of care, 40 percent devoted the equivalent of full-time working hours, plus overtime, to that care (ISR Newsletter, Winter 1977). In addition to direct care, women carry a worry burden. In a recent Canadian study, two-thirds of women over 50 with a living parent said they worried about the parent's health (Marshall, Rosenthal, & Synge, 1983). Several authors suggest that the need for parent-caring (G. L. Lieberman, in press) is changing life in the middle years for many women. Brody (1978) discusses how parents may present a "refilling of the empty nest." Tobin and Kulys (1980) call the view of the empty nest years as a time of carefree personal growth a myth. Increasingly, concerns are expressed that parent-caring may lead to a sense of overload and stress, which may threaten middle-aged women's physical as well as mental health and, in turn, create a bleak outlook for their own old age (Archbold, 1982; Brody, 1982; Robinson & Thurnher, 1979).

Such concerns have also pointed to new needs in the younger generation. It is becoming clear that the state of the economy, as well as mounting divorce rates among young adults, are putting new strains on families. A growing number of mature offspring are now turning to their parents for shelter as well as emotional and financial support.

It is important, however, to look both "up" and "down" generational lines, and to consider the total generational picture in a given lineal unit. The likelihood of the middle generations experiencing a "squeeze" is influenced by the needs and resources of several generations. Valerie Oppenheimer (1981) has given an excellent discussion of how patterns in timing or parenthood in three or more generations will influence the total intergenerational constellation of financial resources, including the probability that the middle generation will experience financial "overload." A similar multigenerational view is necessary if we consider other strains of kinkeeping.

Smith (1983) found that when middle-aged women experienced a sense of overload in caring for aged parents, they tended to have young adult children who were "off track" in *their* life course development. For example, one woman had a son in his late 20s, still without a job; another had a daughter whose marriage had failed and who had moved back into her old room. This study points to the importance of considering support patterns as well as expectations across more than one parent–child link.

It is possible that many women who have heavy parent-caring responsibilities manage this stress because of a supportive relationship "down" generational lines, to a daughter.

EMERGING ISSUES

Finding a Right Balance

As briefly discussed above, a number of authors have warned that strong kin involvement for older women may represent a threat to their physical and mental health. Lehr (1983) draws a parallel to extreme job-centeredness for men, arguing that it causes problems in aging similar to those caused by extreme family centeredness in women. Hess and Waring (1978) discuss "a Goldilocks effect": too much and too little kin involvement seem to have negative consequences. Lehr (1983) and Brody (1982) suggest that legislation and supportive services must be developed to allow women an optimal level of family involvement, one which allows room for them to maintain independent interests and lives. Siegler and George (in press), in a study of life events, have given a new twist to views of women's roles as kinkeeper and family monitor. They found that because of their strong investment in other people's lives, women often mention events that happened to other family members when they are asked to list the best and worst things that happened to them over a given time period. Especially in the case of stressful events, this vicarious involvement in the "ups and downs" of others may leave women with a sense of powerlessness and overload.

Role Ambiguity in Multigenerational Families

Consequences of strong kin involvement have also been discussed with regard to the unprecedented number of multigenerational families. In such families, we are likely to find mothers and daughters aging together. This appears to present some new problems and issues.

In a recent German study, Lehr (1983) put ads in local news-papers, asking members of five-generation families to contact her. She received 340 responses. Exploratory data collection has found a number of families with three generations of widows. Interviews with five generations of women have demonstrated the ambiguity experienced in this situation. It is not at all clear who has the right to some of the privileges of old age, and whose duty it is to ensure them. The interviews often found a strong sense of jealousy in the two generations below the omega. They felt that the omega was receiving all the attention, and they were missing out on some of their returns on earlier family investment. Since some of the great-great-grandmothers were centenarians, the caregiving daughter was herself in advanced old age. Nearly 90 percent of the oldest gener-ation were living in private households, rather than institutions. Among these noninstitutionalized great-great-grandparents, 50 percent lived with a daughter. The German investigators warn that we may see increased rates of illness in young-old women in these families, both because of the stress of caring for the very old and because of possible benefits from the sick role.

Investigators have also begun to ponder what happens to grandparenthood in multigenerational families. At a recent profes-sional meeting, an Israeli researcher described family scenarios where a child called "Grandma," and three women, from three generations, responded. However, I know of no systematic re-search in this area.

Effects of Divorce and Family Reconstitution

Research on kin interaction following divorce points to a possible strengthening of what some authors refer to as "the matrifocal tilt." Since custody goes to the mother in nine out of ten cases, children of divorce are likely to grow up with strong ties to mater-nal kin, and disrupted or weak ties to the paternal family. Pat-terns of remarriage may further reinforce such trends.

When divorced men remarry and start second families, they often have wives who are significantly younger. It is not unusual for men in their 50s and 60s to have young children. Thus, they are becoming fathers at the same time they are becoming grand-fathers in their first family of procreation.

Such family patterns may reinforce the matrifocal tilt for a number of reasons. Children in the second family are likely to know only their maternal grandparents, particularly in the case of the grandfather. As adults, they are likely to experience paternal death "off-time" and spend a disproportionate amount of time with only their mother living. Their children, again, in many cases, will never know their paternal grandfather.

SUMMARY

This chapter has explored older women's involvement in vertical family ties—relationships across generations. It has pointed to the fact that demographic change has created a new intergenerational context for family relationships. With a life expectancy of about 80, women now often spend five to six decades as mothers, and three to four decades as grandmothers. Because of persistent sex differences in early socialization and adult role patterns, the quality of vertical ties in the family are primarily maintained and shaped by women. Their strong, lifelong investment in family ties provides them with a secure base of interpersonal support and continuity. It also opens possibilities for overload and stress, which may threaten their well-being, their mental and physical health, in old age.

Both in the planning and the structuring of individual life paths, and in the development of social policy, members of our aging society are faced with the challenge of maximizing the potential strengths of vertical family ties, yet supporting individual autonomy and personal life space.

11
Adjustment to Family Losses: Grief in Frail Elderly Women

IRENE BURNSIDE

*"Now that my loves are dead
On what shall my action ride?"*

Irene Clarement de Castillejo,
(1973, p. 156)

This chapter focuses on one special segment of older women: frail elderly women. By frail elderly I mean women who are in their 70s, 80s, 90s and centenarians who have high needs in psychosocial, economic, or health areas. Women cope with many losses in the later years of their lives, but one of the most poignant is loss of family, and/or significant others. This chapter will cover only loss of spouse, loss of children, and loss of significant pets.

Widowhood has not been of great interest to society in spite of its frequency and concomitant problems (Abrahams, 1972). Widows still have to muddle through pretty much on their own. Books by Lynne Caine (1974, 1978) and others have been helpful, but Caine was a young widow and her advice does not address the needs of the frail elderly woman.

CHANGES IN LIFE CYCLE OF WOMEN

The life cycle of women in the United States has undergone dramatic changes in the last 80 years (Block, Davidson, & Grambs,

1981). In 1880 the average woman was widowed young, in fact, before her last child left home. Her last child would be married when she was 55 and she would live to about the age of 68 (Neugarten & Datan, 1973). Now a woman who reaches the age of 65 can expect to live 18 more years on the average, or approximately to an age of 83. The life span of women now may be more than 30 years after the youngest child leaves home (Block et al., 1981). In 1976, eight of every ten older men, but only six of every ten older women lived in a family setting (Special Committee on Aging, 1977).

White women have the longest life expectancy at 78.2 years, followed by black women, 72.7, white men at 70.6, and black men at 64.0. Women are outliving men by approximately eight years and the same approximation holds for both whites and blacks. Widows age 65 and over constitute 31 percent of all people aged 65 years and over and 53 percent of all elderly women (U.S. DHEW, 1976). The average age at which widowhood occurs in America is 56 years (Bengtson, Kasschau, & Ragan, 1977).

Four reasons explain the existence of such a large number of elderly widows (Block et al., 1981):

1. The high mortality rate for males of all ages.
2. Disparity in ages between husbands and wives.
3. The limited opportunity to remarry because of the relatively small number of available males over age 65.
4. The double standard that exists, namely, men may marry women younger than they, but widows are not expected to take husbands who are younger than they are.

Only white men past the age of 75 have a chance of remarrying. The probability is essentially zero for white and black widows and widowers.

It is well established by researchers that there is a connection between emotional and physical reactions. Bornstein, Clayton, Halikas, Maurice, and Robins (1973) showed that those who became depressed during the bereavement period were likely to report a disproportionately higher level of poor health one year later than those who did not report depressive reactions. Several researchers have demonstrated that younger people have more physical symptoms during bereavement than older persons (Clayton, 1975; Maddison & Viola, 1968; Parkes, 1972).

Gerber, Rusalem, Hannon, Battin, and Arkin (1975) found

that older widows who experienced an extended period of grief, and anticipated grief prior to the spouse's death, did not adjust to the loss any better than those who faced a sudden loss.

Research shows that younger persons have more physical symptoms in bereavement, but there is one common complaint among elderly widowed women: that they do not get used to the state of widowhood. In Lopata's Chicago study (1973) about widows, 48 percent stated they had gotten over their husbands' death within a year; about 20 percent said they had never gotten over it, and did not expect to. As one widow once said to me, "I have gotten over it, but I have not gotten used to it." Silverman (1974) states that the widow acts as if she were still her husband's wife. She does not think of herself as a widow and that may last as long as one month.

Some women who have lost husbands have a large network of other widows that help them through the experience. Some have widowed sisters or other women relatives who rally around them. Neighbors often can be tremendously helpful during the time of grief. Parkes states that widows suffer from loss, stigma, and deprivation. The loss leads to grief; the stigma leads to altered self-concept and isolation; the deprivation leads to poignant loneliness (Parkes, 1972).

Arling (1976:84) concluded in his study that friends and neighbors are a better resource than family for avoiding isolation in later life. Does this finding have implications for health care professionals working with elderly women?

The following is an example of a widow who moved across country.

CASE EXAMPLE I

Mrs. C. is 86 years old. She had always been a housewife and had only an eighth grade education. She had been married for 60 years and had moved only two times during the entire 60 years. She had lived most of her adult life in the same house with her husband. A third move occurred about 5 years after her husband died. She was 71 years old at that time and felt that the house on the East Coast was too large for her to take care of. She sold the house and got rid of her many possessions and moved to California to be near her sister, five years older than she. Mrs. C. said this was her last sibling and she felt she wanted to be with her. The sister became increasingly feeble and Mrs. C. could not take care of her in their condominium. The sister moved in with one of her grandchildren. Mrs. C. had no children and once again she was alone, but this time in a modern condominium instead of her large rambling old Southern home. She was without friends she had known for many years and the support of her neighbors. She adjusted quite well in spite of the tremendous move. She was in fairly good health, although she lightened her volunteer work when she suffered from some angina. She spends time weekly in a thrift shop as a volunteer. There she meets women with similar lifestyles and the volunteer work gives meaning to her life. It is interesting that she never had children of her own, but she is in charge of children's clothing in the thrift shop. She continues to do her own sewing and she knits sweaters. She dresses smartly and drives her own car. She does not seem to feel sorry for herself, but does sound a bit wistful when she says, "I miss my house and all my friends back in Virginia from time to time."

Some of the frail elderly women who move during the bereavement period move great distances to be closer to families. Sometimes they move to be with relatives they never were very close to in the first place, or as in this instance they move and end up having to care for someone else. Two other women I know moved halfway across the country to be near nephews whom they were not particularly close to. In one instance, the woman subsequently had a stroke and the nephew immediately took over her possessions and made all of her decisions, even though she knew what was happening; she could not write or speak well. The other woman is unhappy and does not like the climate of the new state or the new community. She left all of her professional friends and former co-workers behind, and has been unable to make new friends easily.

The minute a frail older woman shows some signs of forgetfulness or not being as sharp as she once was, she becomes vulnerable. We all know of instances when a relative or children move in and take over and literally pull the rug out from under the older woman. A feisty older woman also may be seen as out of character and ill as in the following example related by Judith Agee (1980).

CASE EXAMPLE II

A psychiatrist was called for a consultation to a home for the aged because an elderly woman wished to divorce her husband. The couple were in their 80s. They had resided in the home for several years. They had been married for 60 years. The wife was considered to be mentally ill. Her children were quite upset about the mother and her determination to be divorced so they requested a psychiatric consultation. When the psychiatrist asked her about wanting the divorce after 60 years of marriage, raising children, and a life together with one man, she replied, "Enough is enough."

While this is not an example of grief work and bereavement, it is an example of the expectations that are set up for older women and the commotion that can be created when they do not fit into the expectations or roles that others have for them. And that, of course, is a common and recurring problem.

Gordon Streib (1975) makes the point that in the future, there will be an increase in the number of women who have experienced divorce at some time in their lives and will have already had a rehearsal for how it is to live alone.

And Chevan and Korson (1972, p. 46) make a salient point that living alone is not synonymous with social isolation: "Maintenance of an independent household is for many of the widowed the symbolic bastion within which they define their roles. To think of living any other way is abhorrent, entailing a loss of privacy as well as independence, and thereby threatening the integrity of personal adjustment." The same researchers found that better educated women are more likely to be living alone, and also those with more income. They are also likely to be younger, for at the age of 80 or more, the maintenance of a household does become arduous because of increased physical limitations and/or lowering of the energy level.

One of the ways that older women may cope with their grief is to "sanctify the memory," a term used by Troll, Miller, and Atchley (1979, p. 71). In this intellectual process, all of the negative characteristics are erased and the person retains only a very positive, idealized memory of the deceased. This reminds one of the work of Eric Lindemann (1944) when he described one of the tasks of grief work as developing and cultivating an acceptable memory or image of the deceased. Troll, Miller, and Atchley (1979) state it well: "Somehow we think it wrong to speak ill of the dead." But widows not only do not speak ill, they truly do not think ill and even tend to exaggerate or make up good qualities (p. 71). These authors feel that idealization of the dead can have a positive value in that it satisfies the need of the survivor to believe that each life has some meaning. Lopata (1973) points out that it could interfere with the formation of new intimate relationships; if one's dead spouse was so ideal, no living human could match him.

Some of the elderly women I have known said that living alone has helped them to prepare for dying, for they realize that dying is something they will do alone. And although some persons abhor the thought of living alone, there are others who handle it well. One octogenarian, a Jungian analyst, wrote about living alone during her widowhood. Florida Scott-Maxwell (1968, p. 33) wrote,

> I wonder if living alone makes one more alive. No precious energy goes
> in disagreement or compromise. No need to augment others. There is just
> yourself, just truth—a morsel—and you. You went through those long
> years when it was pain to be alone, now you have come out on the good
> side of that severe discipline.

Another type of grief, anticipatory grief, is appearing more frequently in the aging women who are caring for a spouse who has senile dementia, or the more preferred diagnosis, Alzheimer's disease. Frail women are caring for men who are confused, wandering, suffering from Sundowner's syndrome, and in the later stages may not recognize the wife. The nonrecognition is particularly devastating to the spouse caring for them.

CASE EXAMPLE III

A woman in her late 70s cared for a husband in his 80s during the early stages of Alzheimer's disease. She accepted the burden of care willingly and was coping fairly well. She went off to a bridge game with some of her friends and came home late one night. She had forgotten her key and when her husband opened the door he did not recognize her and shouted unkind words at her and slammed the door in her face. This was one of the very difficult times for her. At times like these, the frail elderly woman needs much support and caring herself.

HALLUCINATIONS IN WIDOWHOOD

Rees studied 253 widowed persons in England (1971). His findings revealed that young people are less likely to hallucinate than those widowed after the age of 40. Almost half of the people interviewed had hallucinations of the dead spouse. These episodes were most common during the first ten years of widowhood. Social isolation did not affect the incidence of hallucinations and it was not related to depressive illness. There was no variation within cultural group nor in the place of residence. Most subjects (68.6%) perceived the hallucinations as helping them. The hallucinations occurred at variable times throughout the day, and in what appeared to be a normally healthy sample of persons. The senses involved were vision, hearing, and touch.

I consider this to be an important study because most of us in the health care field do not consider hallucinations as normal or helpful. Perhaps we need to reconsider and evaluate the concept of hallucinations and study them further, especially in regard to the elderly bereaved (Burnside, 1982).

ANOTHER POIGNANT LOSS:
LOSS OF ONE'S CHILDREN

In *The Old Ones of New Mexico* by Robert Coles (1975: p. 10) is this lovely passage by an old woman:

> I thought of the five children we had lost, three before they had a chance to take a breath. I wondered where in the universe they were. In the evening sometimes, when I go to close loose doors that otherwise complain loudly all night, I am likely to look at the stars and feel my long-gone infants near at hand. They are far off, I know, but in my mind they have become those stars—very small, but shining there bravely, no matter how cold it is far up. If the stars have courage, we ought to have courage; that is what I was thinking, as I so often have in the past.

In one nursing home a woman in her 80s who had been widowed and only had one child was informed that her son had been killed in an automobile accident. The staff members dreaded having to tell her, and they were concerned how she would handle the tragic news since she was already struggling with many health problems of her own. A friend in a wheelchair wheeled herself into the room and asked if she would like for her just to sit with her for awhile. The grieving woman said she would like that and so a group of women were enlisted by this friend to rotate for half hour periods (their own energy levels were low; remember they were also in wheelchairs) and they sat quietly at her bedside conversing only when she wished it.

The solutions that older women can come up with are sometimes so superior to those we care takers have that it is surprising that we do not consult them more often. In fact, Gordon Streib (1975) stated something similar when he wrote,

> It will be to the advantage of our older citizens to see what they can do
> for each other to make their daily lives happier—to improve their micro-
> environment. And because women are healthier, longer-lived, and have
> special abilities of organizing, or socializing and caring, I predict that
> they will take the lead in improving the life style of America's older
> citizens in the future.

I would only add that they will also show us the many ways to bear grief and sadness.

SIGNIFICANT PETS

Thus far, this chapter has focused on loss of spouse and loss of a child. We have not any systematic studies of the impact of pets on those elderly who have been attached to pets and lost them. We do know that studies reveal survival effects that are related to companion pets (Friedman, 1979). The pets can be cats or dogs, or budgies as a study in Wales showed. There is now a new society for promotion of study and understanding of the human/animal bond called The Delta Society. Bustad, a veterinarian (1980, p. 125) reminds us,

> For old people, too often in the family and especially outside the family,
> attention and love are not common commodities. Companion animals
> may be a significant part, and in some cases, the only source of warmth,
> affection, love and devotion for the elderly. Pets seem to negate some of
> the unfortunate health effects of the stresses of living. For many cases,
> pets give people a good reason for living.

Bustad (1982, personal communication) has also shared that people show up in veterinary offices with healthy pets. The vet examines the animal but cannot find anything wrong with the pet, but as the owner begins to talk, the owner reveals a loss or emotional suffering and spends the time discussing the loss or the sadness being experienced. Bustad and Hines (1982) ask an important question: "At what period in a person's lifespan will possession of an animal companion have the most influence?" I would suggest that during grief work is one very important time.

The following is a case example of the importance of the human/animal bond. It occurred in Los Angeles some years ago.

CASE EXAMPLE IV

Mrs. B. was in her late 70s. She had been a buyer for a large department store in Los Angeles. She had been married but had no children. Her husband left her for a younger woman and after she was divorced, she moved into a hotel in the downtown area and lived frugally. She took excellent care of her expensive clothes, which were purchased when she worked and she was smartly dressed in spite of a very low income. She had been given a puppy as a birthday present by her husband. She and the old dog lived together in the rundown hotel. When the dog, who by then was 17 years old, died, she could not bear to bury it and kept it in the apartment until it began to decompose. Then she covered it with blankets and laid it outside of her door in the hallway. The public health department was promptly called and she was taken off to a psychiatric unit. A young conservator, who was studying law, was assigned to her. When she went to the hotel, she found that the woman in a last moment of rage had thrown a plant to the floor and broken it. The conservator gathered up the plant, bought a new pot and repotted the plant and helped the woman resettle in a new location. The conservator felt that the plant incident was symbolic of the tremendous loss she was experiencing and how her world was truly falling apart. She befriended her, helped her move her possessions, and helped her readjust to the new living situation.

Not infrequently does one hear of women wrapping a dead pet bird in foil and placing it in the deep freeze. One of my neighbors did just that with her mynah bird. When her two small grandchildren came to visit, they found the bird in the deep freeze when they were looking for popsicles. One little boy turned to the other and said, "Do you suppose she will do that to Grandpa when he dies?"

It is recommended by Dr. Bustad that when a pet is ailing and will need to be put to sleep or will die, another pet be introduced to take its place before the original pet is gone. We do not very often think of the importance of significant pets, but health care givers are now beginning to realize the importance of assessing those relationships also.

To pull all of this together, I have extrapolated some guidelines from the literature which might be helpful for those caring for older frail women. These guidelines come from a variety of sources and disciplines. Because each woman is different and unique, an individual approach, of course, will be needed. Perhaps this last will alert the caregiver. That is its intent: to prepare us and to make us more sensitive and thoughtful about the needs of the frail elderly women doing grief work.

Grief for a Spouse

- Grief work is individual and may be expressed in a variety of ways; we need to respect the method or way an elderly woman chooses to work through her grief and bereavement and pain.
- Not all elderly women are grieving after a husband dies. A few have shown tremendous relief that their life of hardship and the endurance struggle is over. Some even blossom and flourish when they are alone.
- One of the major tasks of widowhood is identity reconstruction (Lopata, 1975). We will need to help widows move in that direction. Sometimes women who have never had a chance to attend college have returned to school. In their 70s and 80s they attain a goal once denied them. Some universities offer special tuition fees, or even centers to rest, study, and relax for the students beyond age 65.
- Grief work for a widow can last from a year to a lifetime.
- Widows usually resist moving to the homes of married children (Loether, 1975). They may need assistance in maintaining their own independent living quarters.
- Elderly women caring for terminally ill spouses may neglect their own health during the time of caring for the partner. For instance, in Alzheimer's disease, the widow should be assisted in finding a support group. Not only

are older women caring for husbands, but sometimes a woman in her 80s will be caring for a child in his or her 60s who has Alzheimer's disease. To continue in such difficult, strenuous caretaking roles, they will need support and assistance so their own health is not impaired. *The 36 Hour Day,* a book by Nancy Mace and Peter Rabins (1981), is highly recommended.

- Many women make internal preparations and role play in themselves the prospect of widowhood (Rosow, 1967). This may be an adaptive task that we have not encouraged enough in health care.
- Older women may be reluctant to take on the responsibilities that a new marriage would require (Treas & VanHilst, 1976).
- Older widows may be high users of outpatient clinics.
- Grief cannot be hurried up. Sad memories may be evoked by music, pictures, etc. Time should be spent listening.
- Women may take an item of the deceased husband and wear it for a long time. It could be a bathrobe, a jacket, a shirt, some item that helps them feel close to the deceased. Therefore, relatives should be discouraged from hastily throwing things out or giving them away.
- Hallucinations after the death of a spouse are common. Survivors in one study, according to Rees, found them helpful.
- We need to better understand the concept of hallucinations and the important role they play in grief work of elderly women.
- Encourage the life review as Butler has suggested, so the widow can come to grips with her own life, his life, and their life together (Butler, 1963).
- Listen to the details of the funeral, the events prior to the funeral as the older woman replays it. It may require great patience to be that listener.
- Try to understand how grief work in the older woman might be different from grief work in the young woman.

Morgan (1976) advises us to look at the problems which accompany widowhood rather than viewing widowhood as a problem. That is good advice.

Grief for a Child

- Anniversaries of death and birthdays are sometimes not recognized as a cause for sadness in the elderly woman. You might need to ask about such dates and times and help the aged woman acknowledge the cause of the present sorrow (Gramlich, 1968).
- Peers can be most helpful in the grief work and they should be encouraged to help in their roles with friends who grieve.
- Older women will remember for years and years a child she has lost, even a stillborn or a miscarriage. If she needs to talk about it, practice active listening during these times.
- Older women will also grieve for older children who have died. Do not be surprised if a woman says, "If he had lived, he would now be 65 years old."
- It is particularly painful for an adult parent to lose an adult child.

Grief for a Pet

- The terminally ill may create difficulties for an aged person. The caregiver may need to assist with the trips to the veterinarian, the burial of the pet, and/or the replacement of the animal.
- Watching goldfish or petting animals is beneficial to owners. The importance and the psychological health involved in pet ownership should not be discounted by relatives or caregivers who themselves may be prejudiced against pet ownership.
- Assessing the health status of the pet may be important for the caregiver. Reduced care and/or neglect of an animal may be an indication that the older woman cannot cope with her caring responsibilities anymore. For example, one woman on a psychiatric unit was admitted because she was feeding her canary a can of dog food every day.
- Pets may be therapeutic during grief. One lonely and isolated woman in her 80s was handling her grief with great difficulty and many somatic complaints. A caring neighbor got a puppy for her. Her entire life changed and her motivation and purpose in life increased.

- The use of animals in institutions is now gaining increasing attention. Withdrawn and isolated and depressed older women will respond to a cat or a kitten. One woman in her 90s sits for hours in the lounge area of an Intermediate Care Facility watching the beautiful fish in the fish tank. She says it makes her feel peaceful inside.

I should like to end my chapter with this short poem by Carl Sandburg (1970, p. 49).

Give me a hunger,
O you gods who sit and give
The world its orders.
Give me hunger, pain and want. . . .
But leave me a little love,
A voice to speak to me in the day end,
A hand to touch me in the dark room
Breaking the long loneliness.

RESOURCES

Films

Lila, 16 mm, 29 minutes. Lila Bonner-Miller would appear to be an ordinary lady; she's a leader in her church, loves plants and cooking, and is a great-grandmother. But at 80 years of age, she is also a psychiatrist who continues to practice, often using art as therapy. Lila was a member of the first class at the University of Virginia to admit women to its medical school. Contact: Ideas and Images, P.O. Box 5354, Atlanta, GA 30307.

Keeping Going, video, 26 minutes. Beth Harrison is a 78-year-old widow who lives alone in a small trailer park in a mountain area north of Santa Cruz, California. She is partially blind and suffers from severe arthritis. She maintains her independence through special community support services. She is shown at her daily round of activities and her participation in the Senior Health Maintenance Program, including nursing assessment, group health education, and the community health volunteer program. Contact:

William J. McEwen, Ph.D., Consultant in Behavioral Sciences, California Department of Health Services, 871 Santa Barbara Road, Berkeley, CA 94707.

World of Light: A Portrait of May Sarton, 16 mm or video, 30 minutes. This film on the life of a writer is photographed in the New England areas where Sarton lives. The artistic touch is evident everywhere in the rich and lush colors. Contact: ISHTAR, 305 East 11th Street, New York, NY 10003.

Chillysmith Farm, 16 mm, 55 minutes. This is a ten-year documentation of a family confronting stereotypes as they grapple with old problems while searching for new answers. The film was inspired by the award-winning book *Gramp;* the film recalls Gramp's story. His wife, Nan, recounts the family's intergenerational experience with aging and dying. Contact: Filmmakers Library, Inc., 133 East 58th Street, Suite 703A, New York, NY 10022, (212) 355-6545.

Organizations

Delta Society, N.E. 1705 Upper Drive, Pullman, Washington 99163. Professional association to promote the health and well-being of people and animals by investigating the relationship between them and with their environment.

12
Poverty and Minority Status

JACQUELYNE JOHNSON JACKSON

Three major problems that hinder a reasonable consideration of the vulnerabilities and strengths of women who are old, poor, and members of racial minorities are elucidated in this chapter. *Old* is defined conveniently as over 65 years of age, notwithstanding the well-recognized and accepted fact that some people who are quadruply jeopardized by their sex, age, income status, and race may be functionally old before they become chronologically old. The first problem concerns operationalizations of the concepts of poverty and of minority status and extends to a consideration of the erroneous equating of racism to sexism or ageism. The second deals with double jeopardy and with purported tests of that hypothesis. The third simply considers globally the status of available data about quadruply jeopardized people, illustrated best by a limited focus upon comparative mortality data for old black and white women and men.

Most of the illustrations given are about old, black women, primarily because quadruple jeopardy was coined specifically to refer to poor, old, black women (J. Jackson, 1971). Also, most old women classified as a racial minority are black. In 1981, of all old women in the United States, 90.7 percent were white and 8.2 percent were black (U.S. Department of Commerce, 1982b). Further, most of the few empirical data available about quadruply jeopardized people pertain only to blacks.

OPERATIONALIZING POVERTY

Ethnogerontologists, most of whom study aged minorities in the United States, typically operationalize poverty by accepting the

166

federal definition or by arbitrarily defining it to fit their survey data. In using aggregated data collected by federal agencies, the definition of poverty relied upon is usually that developed by the Federal Interagency Committee. It typically adjusts the poverty level by changes in the Consumer Price Index, where the resulting poverty levels are generally based upon total money income instead of a combination of cash and in-kind subsidies, such as food stamps, housing, and Medicaid. But any feasible determination of the poverty level of the aged must be based upon cash and in-kind subsidies; otherwise the poverty rate of the aged is overestimated (Snyder, 1979).

Identification of the category of quadruply jeopardized people, one element of which is their income status, is impossible without data about their total real income. As an example, an arbitrary definition of poverty, for a comparison of aged blacks and whites in a secondary data set, is illustrated by J. Jackson and Walls (1978). They dichotomized low-income and high-income aged subjects in the 1974 Harris survey (National Council on Aging, Inc., 1976) on the basis of 1973 household income as under and over $4000. In that instance, to have done otherwise would have prohibited any statistically meaningful comparisons between aged blacks and whites of grossly similar income statuses. In 1973, the median household income of all races in the United States was $10,512 and, for blacks $6485 (U. S. Dept. of Commerce, 1982b).

Such studies as those focused upon the feminization of poverty, racial comparisons of poverty rates of the aged, or even comparisons of the social characteristics of poor and nonpoor black women who are old, all require realistic or concrete definitions of poverty. Under most currently operationalized definitions, as indicated above, some people defined as poor actually have higher total real incomes than do those defined as nonpoor. Take the cases of Mrs. Poor and Mrs. Rich, as of 1983.

Hypothetically, Mrs. Poor's cash income of $2057 in 1983 was at the poverty level, but it was supplemented by $4028 in in-kind subsidies, totaling $6085. Mrs. Rich, a resident of the same central city, had a total real income of $5877. Ineligible for in-kind subsidies, including Medicaid, Mrs. Rich continued to pay a monthly housing mortgage of $253.83. Who was poorer?

Appropriate classifications of the poverty level status of Mrs. Poor and Mrs. Rich could be improved if ethnogerontologic definitions of poverty level status were based upon total real income instead of cash income. Also, determinations could be based

upon per capita income, following deductions for rental or housing payments, including taxes. The federal definition of poverty
for a single individual could then be employed to determine
whether a given individual was above or below the poverty level
for the applicable year. Judgments would be based upon per capita
income minus the tenure deductions specified above for the year
preceding the administration of the instrument.

OPERATIONALIZING MINORITY STATUS

The classic definition of minority group as "any group of people
who because of their physical or cultural characteristics, are
singled out from the others in the society in which they live for
differential and unequal treatment, and who therefore regard
themselves as objects of collective discrimination" (Wirth, 1945,
p. 347) means that minority group members must experience discrimination and must recognize that they are discriminated
against, or at least so perceive themselves. If quadruply jeopardized people constitute a minority group under this definition,
a definition that clearly also recognizes the power element, they
must perceive themselves as being discriminated against on account of their income status, age, race, and sex. Empirical data
are not yet available to tell us whether people we have characterized as victims of quadruple jeopardy are, in fact, such victims.
Also of some importance is the fact that there is no organization
in the United States devoted to such people. This is especially tell-
ing in a contemporary society with special-interest groups devoted
to almost any and every category of people seeking preferential
treatment.

Thus, we must ask about the theoretical conditions necessary
to justify the labeling of people characterized as being quadruply
jeopardized as a minority group or as possessing minority group
status. Hacker's (1951) distinction between minority group and
minority group status is useful. Minority group status does not
require discriminatory awareness by the victims. Instead, it refers
to people who do not recognize discriminatory group treatment
against them or who accept the propriety of that treatment. So
quadruple jeopardy could be viewed as one form of minority
group status. That status would be based upon the objective, and
not a subjective, determination of that status. Consequently, using
that standard, people who are poor and old and female and members of racial minorities could be determined to hold minority

status, provided that it could be shown conclusively that they are discriminated against on the basis of those four specific characteristics, whether they recognize themselves to be so discriminated against or not.

In the event that empirical data fail to support the labeling of such people as a minority group or as holding minority group status, then consideration should be given to membership they may already hold in one or more minority groups. We have no clear evidence about the manners in which women who are old, poor, and members of a racial minority characterize themselves societally, but impressionistic judgments suggest strongly that most of those now alive would consider themselves to be a minority group member only on account of their racial or ethnic backgrounds. That is, they do not consider themselves as members of any minority based upon sex, age, or income.

One solution to defining minority status may be to follow federal designations of minorities—specifically American Indians, Aleuts, and Eskimos, Asians and Pacific Islanders, Blacks, and Hispanics. But there is growing conflict in various quarters about those designations, especially when certain subgroups included in those classifications have themselves not experienced any substantial or prolonged discrimination in the United States, as in the case of white aliens from Spain. Questions are also being raised about white Cubans. Language or surnames, both mutable traits, may not be sufficient for minority classification.

Perhaps ethnogerontologists should restrict their operationalized definition of minority status to members of groups that have experienced legal discrimination by virtue of their racial or ethnic background in the United States. Some consideration might be given to whether the classification needs to be confined to individuals who were actually in the United States during those years. A counterargument, of course, is that victims of illegal discrimination should not be overlooked. But the main point is that the considerable attempts in recent years to expand greatly the categories of minority groups in the United States have weakened its meaning, and, thereby, its utility and value for sociological inquiries.

RACISM, AGEISM, AND SEXISM

Too many aging professionals tend to draw parallels between racism and sexism or ageism without distinguishing clearly between those "isms." Consider Schaie and Gewitz's (1982, p. 32) claim that

> Discrimination against the elderly simply because of their age is ageism,
> a relatively new -ism that is taking its place among social issues such as
> racism and sexism. . . . Like discrimination on the basis of race or sex,
> ageism in the job market involves rejection of someone as incapable on
> grounds other than the direct assessment of capability.

Many employees are hired without direct assessments of their capabilities. Those capabilities are presumed or inferred from other data. For example, universities generally prefer academicians with terminal degrees because they are presumed to have greater mastery of their disciplines than do their less formally trained competitors. Certain presumptions made in establishing restrictive age qualifications are clearly inapposite for racial qualifications. Assuming that each is in good health for his age, there is a decided difference between the 94-year-old white male and a 24-year-old black male when both are applying for training as a commercial airline pilot and neither has had any previous training or experience with aircraft. Make each male female—the point is the same.

Racism is fundamentally distinct and more invidious than is ageism. Racism is not based upon sexual or gender differences, nor upon such considerations as those of differential response times or the accumulation of physiologic or psychological deficits that accrue with age among older adults. A product of slavery, or certainly its aftermath during the Reconstruction Period, it is based solely on societal and not physiological determinations.

A differentiation between discrimination based on race, sex, or age is apparent in some judicial determinations about employment discrimination. Two applicable statutes are the Civil Rights Act of 1964, Title VII and the Age Discrimination in Employment Act of 1967 (ADEA). Title VII forbids unlawful employment practices against an *individual* due to race, color, religion, sex, or national origin. ADEA forbids such practices against an *individual* who is between 40 and 70 years old on the basis of age in the private sector, but not against an adult in the private sector who is under 40 or more than 70 years of age. In the federal sector, most individuals who are over 40 years of age are covered under ADEA. A review of judicial holdings under Title VII or ADEA indicates that race is not accorded precisely the same treatment as is sex or age (see, e.g., Zimmer, Sullivan, & Richards, 1982). An affirmative defense of bona fide occupational qualification (BFOQ) is available against a claim of employment discrimination based upon sex or age, but not upon race. The BFOQ, of course, must be a legitimate, nondiscriminatory reason (see, e.g., *Dothard v. Rawlinson,* 1977).

Thus, it is reasonable to presume that a nursing home for the aged would not violate Title VII by refusing to hire a male for a position requiring the delivery of intimate, personal services to female patients, but would violate Title VII by refusing to hire an otherwise qualified black female applicant solely on the basis of her race. Further, states are constitutionally prohibited from discriminating against individuals on account of their race, but not on account of their age. In short, the federal courts appear to distinguish somewhat between the immutable trait of race and the mutable trait of age. In social research terms, race is a discrete variable, age is a continuous variable.

OPERATIONALIZING DOUBLE JEOPARDY

The most prevailing theory in the generally atheoretical field of ethnogerontology, an area encompassing minority aging, is double jeopardy and its variants, such as triple or quadruple jeopardy. Double jeopardy was first applied to old blacks, without regard to sex, by Talley and Kaplan (1956). It received limited attention when it appeared in *Double Jeopardy—The Negro in America Today,* a 1964 publication of the National Urban League. Based upon a report from its Detroit affiliate, the League asserted that "Today's aged Negro is different from today's aged white because he *is* Negro. . . . For he has, indeed, been placed in double jeopardy; first, by being Negro and second by being aged" (National Urban League, 1964, p. i). Since then, beginning with J. Jackson's (1967) emphasis on the question of the meaning of being simultaneously old and black, the concept of double jeopardy has enjoyed relatively widespread currency in ethnogerontology and in gerontological circles.

But that concept has also undergone a significant shift in its meaning in certain quarters. For example, Crandall (1980, p. 378) defined jeopardy as referring "to individuals in contemporary society who experience discrimination and prejudice from the society at large because of traits or characteristics that they possess." Crandall (1980) further stated that:

The term "double jeopardy" is applied to individuals who hold two characteristics or traits that the society at large finds undesirable. Many aged individuals are victims of double jeopardy since they possess two characteristics that the society finds undesirable: advanced age and poverty. "Triple jeopardy" refers to individuals who are old, poor, and members of minority groups. "Quadruple jeopardy" refers to individuals who are old, poor, minority-group members, and female. (p. 378)

Crandall does not require any immutable characteristics for double jeopardy. Under his conception, old women who have been unwed mothers and prostitutes could be in triple jeopardy because they possess three societally undesirable traits. His use of double jeopardy distorts its original meaning and illustrates amply the lack of agreement about key concepts in ethnogerontology. Most important, his definition drops an essential element of racial discrimination, an element explicit in the original conception of double jeopardy by Talley and Kaplan (1956).

J. Jackson's (1971) coinage of "quadruple jeopardy" to refer specifically to women who were black, old, and poor contained the essential element of a jeopardizing status due to racial background. Extending the concept to incorporate old and poor women who are not black raises some questions. For example, is it reasonable to include old and poor women who are of Cuban ancestry and racially classified as white under this conception? Should old and poor women, racially classified as white, who are recent immigrants from Peru and who speak little or no English be included?

In *Soberal-Perez v. Schweiker,* United States District Court, Eastern District of New York (1982), the plaintiffs claimed that they were denied equal access to and meaningful participation in the disability and Supplemental Security Insurance programs operated by the Social Security Administration because notices about those programs in Spanish were insufficient and because there were too few Spanish-speaking personnel to serve them. Citing from *Frontera v. Sindell,* 522 F.2d at 1220, the court held that "Our laws are printed in English and our legislatures conduct their business in English." The presumption was that the current procedures of the Social Security Administration applicable to *Soberal-Perez* were racially and ethnically neutral and not subjected to strict scrutiny on a constitutional basis. This decision, subject to appeal at this writing, could be used to argue strongly that at least one element of double or multiple jeopardy should be applicable to strict scrutiny on constitutional grounds. That is, an individual classified by ethnogerontologists as being in double or multiple jeopardy should also be a member of a class held to be suspect under judicial interpretations of the Fourteenth Amendment to the Constitution of the United States.

At least two other problems arise in a consideration of the expansion or contraction of the double jeopardy concept. Briefly, one deals with restrictions to native-born citizens and the other with restrictions based upon socioeconomic status. Restriction to native-born citizens gets around the inclusion of old people who are recent immigrants to the United States and were not subjected to lifelong victimization within the United States on account of their race, but it does not deal adequately with naturalized citizens with lengthy years of residence in the United States. Restrictions based upon the socioeconomic status of a minority group as compared to that of whites could exclude, for example, Japanese Americans from inclusion under double jeopardy; but the original conception of double jeopardy did not focus upon socioeconomic status. That is, being poor or belonging to a group whose overall socioeconomic status was lower than that of whites was not then a conceptual element.

Perhaps the most troublesome problem with double jeopardy is that it has been applied to groups without regard to their considerable heterogeneity. Double jeopardy may well be a time-bound concept. Presented only two years after the U.S. Supreme Court had begun its attack upon the long-prevailing doctrine of "separate, but equal," Talley and Kaplan's (1956) use of it predates such statutory acts as the Civil Rights Act of 1964 and the Voting Rights Act of 1965. It also is a concept that disregards entirely the subjective feelings about, for example, being old and black among those who are, in fact, old and black. Consequently, it may well be more useful as a polemical concept for advocates for aged minorities than for theoretical purposes for ethnogerontologists.

TESTING DOUBLE JEOPARDY

Very few researchers have undertaken empirical tests of double jeopardy and none have used any longitudinal data, as illustrated by M. Jackson and Wood (1976), M. Jackson, Kolody, and Wood (1982), and Dowd and Bengtson (1978). Focusing upon their purported testing of the hypothesis sheds some light on the inherent difficulties of the concept itself.

M. Jackson and Wood (1976) claim to have tested double jeopardy by using data from the 1974 Harris survey on aging. But their research scarcely constituted such a test (J. Jackson & Walls, 1978). Among other problems, they merely regarded racial differences as being significant whenever the percentage gap between blacks and whites on any given item exceeded 10 percent. They employed no statistical tests to determine the significance of differences.

J. Jackson and Walls (1978), who also used the Harris data, did not test double jeopardy, nor was that an intent of their study. Using, where appropriate, weighted Ns to accommodate the oversampling in the Harris survey, they simply compared blacks and whites over 65 years of age and, in separate analyses, blacks and whites between 18 and 64 years of age. Largely using chi-square and t, their tests of significance typically showed no substantial differences by race among the aged. When differences did appear, further analyses were done by controlling for 1973 household income. Extremely few of the variables in the secondary data set distinguished between aged blacks and whites on the basis of race. J. Jackson and Walls were quite aware of the futility of attempting to test the concept of double jeopardy with cross-sectional data involving a heterogeneous grouping of aged blacks.

M. Jackson, Kolody, and Wood (1982, p. 77) proposed "that the situation of older blacks is best characterized as one resulting from the combined effects of age and race." Again using data from the 1974 Harris survey, *double jeopardy* referred to differences between younger whites and aged blacks, *race jeopardy* to differences between aged blacks and whites, and *age jeopardy* to differences between younger and aged blacks. Younger people were between 18 and 39 years of age and older people over 65 years of age. Still relying upon mere percentage differences to determine statistical significance, the researchers concluded that aged blacks were doubly jeopardized by income, health, and life satisfaction. Here, double jeopardy involves comparisons between different races and age cohorts. Some doubt may be raised about the feasibility of that kind of comparison, particularly when it also involves life satisfaction. Also, one would expect the overall health status of younger persons to be better than that of older persons. When that phenomenon occurs, to characterize it as jeopardizing tends to ignore the normal processes of aging, as if they should not occur biologically.

Schaie, Orchowsky, and Parham (1982) used life satisfaction as a dependent variable in illustrating the interacting effect of race on cohort and period effects. Their analyses of data from two national surveys conducted by the National Opinion Research Center in 1973 and 1977 showed

> substantial cohort effects in life satisfaction favoring earlier-born cohorts regardless of race, even when state of health and income was controlled. However, there were significant race differences with respect to period effects, with life satisfaction remaining stable for whites, but increasing for blacks over the period studied. (Schaie, Orchowsky, & Parham, 1982, p. 229)

M. Jackson, Kolody, and Wood (1982) did not compare life satisfaction by controlling for health and income, nor did they employ the kind of methodological analysis used by Schaie, Orchowsky, and Parham (1982), despite the availability of data from the 1980 Harris survey. Thus, the question remains: how do you test feasibly and reasonably the hypothesis of double jeopardy?

Dowd and Bengtson (1978) also attempted to test double jeopardy by using cross-sectional survey data collected from a probability sample of 413 blacks, 449 Mexican Americans, and 407 whites between 45 and 74 years of age, all of whom were residents of Los Angeles County. Their sample was not described by nativity and its ethnic proportions failed to match their distribution within their country.

Dowd and Bengtson (1978:427) defined double or multiple jeopardy as referring "to the additive negative effects of being old *and* black (or any other racial/ethnic minority) on frequently cited indicators of quality of life, such as income, health, housing, or life satisfaction."

Using a complex operationalized definition of double or multiple jeopardy, Dowd and Bengtson (1978:434) concluded that their data

> only partially support those who argue that the world of the minority is one of double jeopardy. Differences in old age across race lines on income or health, for example, do suggest that older blacks and Mexican Americans suffer from a double jeopardy. However, on variables measuring frequency of familial contact, the mean figures for black and Mexican American respondents indicates [*sic*] fairly stable interaction—not less—across each age strata [*sic*]. The existence of double jeopardy,

therefore, is an empirical, not a logical, question. To assume otherwise
would be to ignore the warning of [Donald] Kent . . . that "age may be
a great leveler with regard to both racial and social influences. . . ."

However, since they employed only cross-sectional data, they
could not determine whether a significant decline occurred in the
dependent variable of given subjects as their age increased. An
inference from Schaie, Orchowsky, and Parham (1982) is that
life satisfaction scores of younger blacks are inappropriate prox-
ies for earlier life satisfaction scores of older blacks because
they represent different cohorts. Further, the conception of
double jeopardy by Dowd and Bengtson (1978) ignores entirely
"what might have been" the life achievements or styles of older
blacks had they not lived under conditions of legally sanctioned
racial segregation. The poem never penned, the dream always
deferred can have impact upon judgments of life satisfaction.

Additionally, innumerable questions could be raised about
using primary group interaction as a test of double jeopardy.
Clearly, it would be necessary to show that racial discrimination
is significantly related to primary group interaction prior to using
it as a variable in examining the hypothesis of double jeopardy.
For aged blacks of yesterday and today, one could note that much
of their social gathering on an informal level took place within
their residences, primarily because they were denied entry into
commercial establishments. Also, there is no reason to believe that
race *per se* is a critical determinant of familial or kinship interaction. Consequently, one may readily agree with Dowd and Bengtson (1978) that double jeopardy represents an empirical question,
but one must still contend that its conceptualization is dependent
upon logical and realistic premises. In the latter instance, Dowd
and Bengtson (1978) failed.

That is, the theoretical development of double jeopardy or
multiple jeopardy must be approached logically, provided that the
resulting theory is ultimately testable. Based upon Turner's (1978)
distinction between axiomatic and causal process formats of theoretical construction, the latter is probably more feasible for ethnogerontology. It

> involves an effort to trace the causal sequence of events that influence
> a particular occurrence. Explanation does not involve logical deductions,
> but rather statements of causal connections among variables in a se-
> quence which accounts for the variation in the particular occurrence of
> interest to an investigator. (Turner, 1978:9-10)

Tracing the causal sequences of jeopardizing events influencing the social conditions of old age requires some form of longitudinal methodology, preferably beginning at birth. Such a study would obviously be quite costly, necessitating thereby some further consideration of its feasibility, a consideration not lying within the scope of this chapter. If such a study is ever undertaken, however, cohort comparisons focused merely upon the demographic aggregated groups will be insufficient to determine the effects of a lifelong exposure to racism on the social conditions and life satisfaction of old blacks.

INADEQUATE DATA ABOUT QUADRUPLE JEOPARDY

The scant literature available about quadruply jeopardized people is too fragmented and inconclusive to provide any adequate description and analysis of the consequences of quadruple jeopardy beyond those that may already be envisioned by investigators familiar with demographic comparisons of socioeconomic statuses of racially dominant and racially minority women. A prevailing problem within that literature is the considerable extent to which certain myths about aged blacks are perpetuated. For example, in writing about aged blacks and religion, Carter (1982:107) contended that "because the oppressed person—whether oppression is due to race, class, sex, or age—is forced into a condition of viewing life differently . . . the only source of strength left for the oppressed is his trust in an unseen, just higher power." Aside from his failure to define strength and to support empirically his generalization, Carter (1982) ignored other possibilities of strength for aged blacks, including those who are old and poor women. Many other studies have suggested that the families of both aged blacks and whites often constitute a major source of instrumental and affective support.

In the absence of objectively or subjectively determined quadruple jeopardy, no adequate assessment can be made of the effects of poverty and minority status on living long among old women. But a brief consideration of death rates for aged blacks and whites may be helpful in illustrating further some of the inherent problems in assessing quadruple jeopardy.

J. Jackson's (1982) comparisons of age-adjusted death rates of blacks and whites over 65 years of age, by sex, in the United States, between the years 1964 and 1978, showed that blacks died earlier within each sex group than did whites. The crude death rates showed that the racial crossover in mortality occurred somewhere between 80 and 84 years of age. The likelihood of that crossover within that age-group was waning over time. Among those over 85 years of age, and within each sex group, the racial gap in mortality widened, favoring blacks. The overall socioeconomic status of whites in each of the applicable years was certainly higher than that of blacks, leaving us with the problem of explaining that phenomenon. It is clearly inexplicable by socioeconomic status (J. Jackson, 1982).

Race-sex comparisons of mortality data need to be controlled by socioeconomic data—a massive task. The standard death certificate does contain a space for occupation, but the National Center for Health Statistics does not report deaths by occupation. Often, occupational data on death certificates are either absent or inaccurate. Perhaps appropriate data could be obtained from the files of the Internal Revenue Service, were those files available to investigators. Also, it could be possible for investigators using death certificates to contact relatives or other informants about the deceased, but this is also a time-consuming and expensive project. Yet the need to know the precise relationships between socioeconomic status and death rates is paramount not only for those interested in explaining the phenomenon of racial crossovers in mortality among the aged but also for those interested in conceptualizing and testing an adequate theory of double jeopardy.

In the absence of mortality data controlled by socioeconomic status, an examination of race-sex differences in the suicide rates of the aged may be helpful in that suicide can be considered a surrogate for compounded troubles and zero life satisfaction. The data highlight the fact that the group containing individuals often characterized as being in quadruple jeopardy has the lowest suicide rate. Table 12.1 shows age-adjusted rates for death due to suicide for blacks and whites, by sex, over 65 years of age in the United

TABLE 12.1
Age-adjusted Death Rates due to Suicide per 100,000
of Old Blacks and Whites, by Sex, United States, 1964–1978

Years	Black Women	Black Men	White Men	White Women
1964–1968	1.7	11.0	40.9	8.5
1969–1973	1.8	10.8	39.9	8.9
1974–1978	2.2	13.4	39.4	8.5

States in 1964–1968, 1969–1973, and 1974–1978. As is readily apparent, the rates are lowest for black women in each of the three time periods, followed by white women, black men, and white men. Of greater interest, perhaps, is the increase between the first and third time periods in the black rates, but not in the white rates.

Table 12.2, which contains crude death rates and age-adjusted death rates due to suicide for old blacks and whites in the year 1979, shows that the rates continued to be lowest for black women. Between 1974–1978 and 1979, however, the age-adjusted rate for whites of both sexes and black men declined, whereas that for black women rose somewhat, from 2.2 to 2.5 per 100,000. Also, an examination of the crude death rates for specific age intervals confirms the general increase in suicide rates with increasing age only for white men with a general decrease by age for white women, and a mixed pattern for both black women and men. In 1979, among old black women those between 65 and 69 and between 80 and 84 years of age had the highest suicide rates. How does quadruple jeopardy relate to those rates? We do not know, but we do need answers.

What may be most apparent, perhaps, from the suicide rates presented above is that quadruple jeopardy, objectively defined, may not be very useful, or useful at all, in understanding individual aging, even among old women who are black and poor. Neither do the data about racial crossovers in mortality rates in the very late years of life support strongly an objectively determined notion of quadruple jeopardy. An examination of mor-

TABLE 12.2
Crude and Age-adjusted Death Rates per 100,000
due to Suicide of Old Blacks and Whites by Sex, United States, 1979

Rate	Black Women	Black Men	White Men	White Women
Crude Death Rate				
65–69 years	3.1	13.0	31.5	8.3
70–74 years	1.9	14.2	35.9	7.2
75–79 years	2.1	9.3	46.4	7.2
80–84 years	3.2	13.0	51.0	5.9
85+ years	1.0	15.4	50.2	5.0
Age-adjusted rate				
65+ years	2.5	12.8	37.7	7.5
(1940 Standard Population)				

tality rates in the earlier years of life indicates that those who are victimized by both their race and sex, as opposed to those who may be victimized only by their sex, die much more rapidly during their younger years. Thus, at least some members of a subgroup of the aged classified as being in quadruple jeopardy on the basis of their sociodemographic traits may not, in fact, subjectively consider themselves to be so victimized and it may be in error to suggest that their failure to realize or to accept their status as defined by social scientists places them in the category of minority group status.

SUMMARY

We have come almost full circle to our starting point. Any consideration of the effects of poverty and minority status upon the vulnerabilities and strengths of old women as they relate to the effects of living long is decidedly premature now, primarily because of theoretical and empirical deficits. Aside from the usual types of losses affecting people who live for a very long time, such as increasing deaths of their relatives and friends and increasing physiological deficits due to normal aging, we know very little, in fact almost nothing, about their vulnerabilities and strengths.

Ethnogerontologists must continue to grapple more carefully and logically with such problems as those related to conceptualizations and operationalizations of poverty, minority status, and double or multiple jeopardy. Much thought needs to be given to the theoretical value of the latter concept, including the extent to which it may be time-bound.

Certainly, whatever double jeopardy blacks may experience in old age as a result of being old and black cannot be tested at all through cross-sectional studies alone. If the concept can be conceptualized adequately, so that it is as least ultimately testable, some further distinction is required between objectively determined and subjectively determined double or multiple jeopardy. For example, the meaning of being old, black, female, and poor cannot be understood without knowing what it means to those who are, in fact, old, black, female, and poor. Even when the concept of double or multiple jeopardy is employed, ethnogerontologists should distinguish clearly between research focused only upon the current sociodemographic conditions of a given subgroup of the aged and their normal or abnormal processes of aging.

The vulnerabilities and strengths of old women who live for a very long time, despite their poverty and minority status, are probably quite vast, but research to date prevents us from knowing definitively what those vulnerabilities and strengths might be, aside from their rather obvious biological elitism. We also do not know whether they differ greatly by their vulnerabilities and strengths from old white women who are poor and live for a very long time.

PART V

INTRODUCTION TO TREATMENT ISSUES

As the previous chapters have demonstrated, health problems loom very large for aged women. Diseases and disabilities are sometimes the critical issue limiting independence. The next three chapters present selected aspects of treatment, first dealing in rather broad perspective with nutrition, then from the more specific point of view of the surgeon, and finally identifying some of the problems physicians encounter in the use of drugs. These types of treatment were selected because of their particular relevance to aged women, whose isolation may entail nutritional deficiencies, whose frailty can lead to fractures requiring surgery at advanced ages, and whose multiple chronic conditions pose the risk of polypharmacy and harmful drug interventions.

Mitchell stresses that nutrition is almost uniquely important as both an etiological and a treatment element among the elderly. She describes the relatively high prevalence of malnutrition in the noninstitutionalized elderly population and points out that deficiencies have been found to be more severe in elderly women than in men.

Several factors contribute to malnutrition, including simple poverty, lack of transportation for shopping, faulty food preferences or habits, and physical changes that diminish interest in and enjoyment derived from food, such as taste deficits and dental problems. Malnutrition may be importantly related to the immune system, to reactive or endogenous depression, and to osteoporosis and subsequent hip fractures. Mitchell suggests that desirable calcium intake to avoid bone loss may be considerably greater than the usual "recommended daily allowance."

Additional problems of importance to the older woman may require further elaboration. Obesity can be a very disabling complication in the elderly arthritic or in the woman with other neuromusculoskeletal disabilities. Weight reduction while maintaining adequate intake of vitamins and minerals is a very challenging task for a sedentary older woman whose pattern of activity involves very little caloric expenditure. Eating habits and dietary patterns may be deep-seated and may have strong cultural origins.

Turning to the more specific questions associated with surgery for older women, Welch presents a thoughtful essay, distilling years of clinical experience and expressing an evident respect for the needs, wishes, and situation of the older woman, to whom surgery may appear quite different than it would to a younger woman. Dr. Welch gives us certain general guiding principles, such as the fact that surgery is well tolerated in the ninth decade of life, due to improved anesthesia and surgical techniques, although operative mortality rises rapidly above the age of ninety. He then gives specific advice and information about the management of eight common surgical problems among elderly women, including fracture of the hip. Dr. Welch cautions us, however, that although surgery can assist in meeting several goals of improved function and freedom from pain, the surgeon cannot be expected to restore complete health. He has some cogent comments on the serious ethical dilemma of preservation of life versus quality of life, and he pays proper heed to the stringent limitations imposed by economic costs. It should be remarked at this point that there have been very extensive efforts in recent years to establish cost/benefit analyses and algorithms or decision-trees as a means of guiding decisions about surgery and other therapeutic interventions. Not many of these studies have dealt specifically with the elderly, and this could be a useful avenue of future investigation.

In the final chapter of this section, Hoppel deals with some specific details of a highly important medical issue. Older women use prescription drugs more than do any other persons in the population. Much of this use and inescapable abuse follows from physicians' recommendations. Practitioners may not be aware of the number and complexity of drug regimens to which the patient has already been subjected. There is clear evidence that the number of drugs prescribed is a major factor leading to poor compliance or noncompliance. As Hoppel points out, the number of adverse drug reactions increases with age, particularly after age 50. Also, there is a great lack of information about specific pharmacokinetics, patterns of drug use, actual frequency of adverse drug reactions, and, again, cost/benefit analyses related to such common problems as the treatment of hypertension in the elderly.

Many of the disabling conditions that make their appearance in the lives of older women, including falls and accidents, can be traced to the careless or inadvertent use of medications. The solitary widow may be lonely and depressed, seek relief of her symptoms from medications of various sorts, have progressive chronic illnesses and disabilities treated with a number of drugs, and, if her mental abilities are failing, be unable to manage accurately a large and complicated drug regimen. Solutions to these problems could range all the way from simple mechanical devices for dispensing medication to refined studies of pharmacokinetics and the behavioral patterns related to illness and disability.

A. B. F.

13
Nutrition as Prevention and Treatment in the Elderly

CAROL O. MITCHELL

There is probably no one single factor that plays such a significant role in contributing to the ultimate health status, general well-being, and quality of life of the elderly woman than does nutrition. Sufficient evidence is available to confirm that one's nutritional habits from childhood throughout adulthood, and on into old age, can predispose one to many of the acute and chronic diseases that are so prevalent in this older age-group.

Not only does nutrition play a role in the etiology of many of these diseases, but it also constitutes a major component of the treatment in a large number of them. Some examples are the low-salt diet in hypertension, the low saturated fat and cholesterol diet in atherosclerosis, the low concentrated sugar diet in diabetes. It has also been postulated that many of the nonspecific symptoms so often encountered in this group may be a result of mild undernutrition. These include mild mental confusion and nervousness, listlessness, anorexia, and the major complaint of being generally tired and weak.

INCIDENCE OF MALNUTRITION

It is estimated that approximately 5 to 10 percent of the noninstitutionalized population over the age of 60 has some degree of malnutrition. Two large national surveys have contributed most to our present knowledge concerning the nutritional status of the elderly. The first was the Ten State Nutritional Survey conducted by the U.S. Department of Health, Education and Welfare in 1968 (U.S. DHEW, 1972). This was a three-year study completed in 1970 focusing primarily on low-income groups because they were considered to be at the highest risk for undernutrition. This study revealed that subjects over the age of 60 consumed diets low in total calories, vitamins A and C, and iron.

The Health and Nutrition Evaluation survey (U.S. DHEW, 1974) was conducted by the National Center for Health Statistics. It encompassed all ethnic and socioeconomic groups and was not limited to one geographic or socioeconomic category. A major finding of this study was that 56.2 percent of the subjects over 60 were consuming diets inadequate in one or more nutrients. Major deficiencies were similar to the findings in the Ten State study. Intakes were low in total calories and protein, along with vitamins A and C, iron, and calcium. Both studies found deficiencies more severe in elderly women than in men.

Adequate data are lacking on the nutritional status of elderly women in nursing homes and other institutions. The few studies available, however, do not indicate that the prevalence of malnutrition is any greater than for the noninstitutionalized. However, it is our experience that only those homes providing high-quality care will even allow such assessments to be made, so the actual incidence may be much higher. The most common form of malnutrition in all populations is subclinical nutritional deficiency, usually involving multiple nutrients characterized by biochemical evidence of reduced tissue levels and/or nutrient-dependent functions (Harrison & Fung, 1982).

Does aging itself alter nutrient needs? A major point of emphasis in gerontology has been that there is great variability among the elderly at any age. Because of the great physiological differences seen, there are also varying nutritional needs in this group. However, the few good studies with very carefully selected subjects of healthy elderly indicate that their nutritional needs do not differ from those of younger adults (Mitchell & Lipschitz, 1982a). One exception is found in the total energy (kilocalorie) needs (National Research Council, 1980). The reduction in energy requirements is based on alterations in body composition, resulting in lower basal metabolic rate (BMR). BMR decreases about 15 to 20 percent between the ages of 30 and 90 years (Shock, 1970). The rate of change in women is less pronounced than that in men because of the higher proportion of body fat and lower BMR of women in young adulthood (Novak, 1972). This lower BMR, coupled with the usual decrease in activity, accounts for the high prevalence of obesity seen in the elderly. Since the requirements for the other macro- and micronutrients do not decline with age, it becomes very important that the diets consumed be of high nutrient density to prevent either the overconsumption of total calories or the underconsumption of other essential nutrients. It must be emphasized that not all elderly subjects decrease their activity level; the energy requirements of these people would not be reduced to the extent usually observed in this group.

FACTORS CONTRIBUTING TO MALNUTRITION

Malnutrition can be caused by any factor that interferes with the process of obtaining, ingesting, digesting, absorbing, or utilizing the essential nutrients. There are a number of social, environmental, and physical factors that often influence the nutritional status of elderly women. An attempt will be made to discuss some of the more important ones.

Probably the most profound problem is the lack of available funds needed to obtain the foods required for an adequate diet. This has always been a problem for the elderly, but in recent years it is affecting more and more of our aged populations, mainly because of the rise in food prices along with the cuts in social programs aimed at providing health care and nutrition services.

Money is not the only reason for poor nutrition among this group. Many elderly persons reject food even when it is available. Older persons living alone may not bother to obtain and cook the food they need even if they have the funds to do so. Therefore, their diet may consist of easy to prepare foods, along with snack foods that are usually high in sugar and low in essential nutrients. Another reason for rejection of food may be the inability to adapt to changes in their lives. These changes are often precipitated from either a loss of a loved one or loss of status resulting from having to give up a position they have held for a significant period of time.

Many elderly people are not physically able to do the shopping required for home meal preparation or they have no access to any type of transportation. The lack of adequate preparation facilities is also often a detriment to providing proper nutrition. This is a particular problem with those elderly women living alone in one room without a refrigerator or stove.

PHYSICAL FACTORS AFFECTING
NUTRITION IN THE ELDERLY

Perceptual ability changes with age. Alterations in taste and smell acuity and, to a lesser degree, changes in sight and hearing, can have a marked influence on patterns of nutrient intake (Busse, 1978). There is considerable controversy as to whether the decline in taste sensitivity seen in older subjects is actually a function of the aging process or is the result of other factors. As with most other alterations seen in the elderly, it is most assuredly multifactorial in origin. A decline in the number of taste buds per papilla has been documented in the elderly, with as much as a 70 percent reduction from age 30 to age 70 years (Hughes, 1969). The taste buds located anteriorly on the tongue are usually the first affected and then progress posteriorly. The affected ones are those that detect sweet or salty quality, leaving those that detect bitter or sour. Nutritional status can also have an influence on the number of taste buds. Several nutrients are known to be important factors for proper cell regeneration to occur. Among these are vitamin A, zinc, vitamin B_{12}, and folate (Kamath, 1982).

It is also known that there is a loss in the ability to detect odors with age. A 68 percent reduction in the sensitivity of the olfactory nerves has been documented, which also has an effect on taste perception (Schiffman, Moss, & Erickson, 1976). These alterations in taste and smell often take some of the pleasure out of eating for these elderly, which may result in less interest in food. It may also help explain many of the complaints that elderly people often have concerning the taste of certain foods.

Oral and dental problems are prevalent in over 50 percent of persons greater than 60 years of age. Poor dentition hinders mastication, which often leads to a lowered food intake along with limiting selection to soft, easy to chew foods. This presumably could lead to a diet deficient in several essential nutrients, particularly good quality protein found in meats and vitamins and minerals from fresh fruits and vegetables.

Another area of controversy is the effect aging has on gastrointestinal function. In aged people, both resting and stimulated secretion of saliva is decreased in volume and in amylose content. This, along with poor mastication, may make it difficult to eat many foods. Decreased activity of some of the other digestive enzymes is also prevalent; however, these are not severe enough to prevent most aged persons from being able to digest a normal diet (Goldman, 1979).

One of the more common gastrointestinal complaints in the elderly is constipation, and the use of laxatives has been found to be twice as great in the above-70 age-group compared to those 40 to 50 years of age. Several factors may contribute to the cause of constipation in older individuals. Among them may be decreased muscle tone and motor function of the bowel, low-fiber diets, inadequate fluid intake, and the ingestion of a number of commonly prescribed drugs. Small changes in eating habits to include more foods high in dietary fiber and increases in fluid intake along with some degree of regular exercise may greatly help to minimize this problem (Harrison & Fung, 1982).

CHRONIC DISEASES AND NUTRITION

Chronic diseases of all types, many of which have a direct impact on diet and nutrition, are more prevalent in the elderly. The management of the disease may include a modified diet that is often hard to follow, either because of the inconvenience of preparation or added expense involved, or it may be unappetizing because of lifelong food preferences. Food intake may also be reduced because of the direct effect the disease or the drugs used to treat the disease has on appetite or nutrient requirement.

Because of the implications of diet in the etiology of certain chronic diseases, nutrition plays an important role not only in their treatment but also in their prevention. Cardiovascular disease is the most prevalent chronic disease state in the elderly. Conflicting evidence exists with regard to whether altering one's dietary habits will reduce the morbidity and mortality of patients with atherosclerotic cardiovascular disease. However, increasing dietary fiber, along with reduction of cholesterol, saturated fat, and salt, has been recommended for young as well as elderly people.

Cancer strikes more people between the age of 60 to 65 years and has the highest mortality rate after the age of 65 (Smith, Bierman, & Robinson, 1978). Loss of appetite, along with the increased metabolic rate makes it difficult for most cancer patients to maintain adequate nutritional status. Aggressive nutritional support of the elderly cancer patient has not been shown to increase survival time. However, evidence is available to suggest that response to treatment as well as quality of life can be improved by maintaining optimal nutritional support in these patients (Lipschitz & Mitchell, 1980).

Osteoporosis, the process resulting from bone mineral loss, has its highest rate of occurrence in white, postmenopausal women. Although extensive research has been performed concerning the mechanism of this bone loss, evidence available regarding this process and its etiology is conflicting (Spencer, Kramer, & Osis, 1982). A decrease in the intestinal absorption of calcium with aging may be one reason for bone loss with age. This has been supported in studies in animals (Hansard, Comar, & Plumlee, 1954), in elderly women (Avioli, McDonald, & Lee, 1965) and in persons over the age of 65 (Bullamore, Gallagher, Wilkinson, Nordin, & Marshall, 1970). Prolonged low intake of calcium has also been implicated; this possibility is supported by the fact that dietary calcium supplementation of one gram daily for one year resulted in significant increases in bone density (44%). The recommended dietary allowance for calcium is 800 mg/day (National Research Council, 1980). Several studies indicate that positive calcium balance cannot be obtained in elderly subjects on this level and that 1200 to 1500 mg/day may be required (Lutwak et al., 1971). Other dietary factors that have been reported to affect calcium status are low intakes of vitamin D and/or fluoride, excess phosphorus intake, and an imbalance of the dietary calcium to phosphorus and calcium to protein intake (Albanese, 1978). In addition to these dietary factors, physical inactivity, hormonal imbalance, and the combined use of alcohol, antacids, and other drugs may also play a role in the balance of bone resorption and synthesis (Spencer et al., 1982).

Anemia has been shown to be significantly higher in the elderly (Hill, 1967; Myers, Saunders, & Chalmers, 1968) and is even more common in low-income blacks (U.S. DHEW, 1972). The anemia is usually attributed either to iron deficiency or to chronic disease, but is not thought to be a normal consequence of aging (R. Lewis, 1976). In most studies, however, there was not sufficient evidence to make a definitive diagnosis of the cause. Lipschitz, Mitchell, and Thompson (1981), in a study of 196 healthy geriatric females, found a high prevalence of anemia. However, after careful hematological evaluations, the etiology of the anemia in all but five of the anemic subjects could not be ascribed to the commonly recognized causes. After further investigations, they suggested that the mechanism of the unexplained anemia was a general reduction in hematopoietic cell numbers, resulting in an overall decrease in hematopoietic reserve. It was further surmised that the presence of anemia may provide a clue to those subjects at greatest risk of an inadequate response to stress.

NUTRITIONAL SUPPORT OF THE MALNOURISHED ELDERLY PATIENT

Recent studies indicate that protein calorie malnutrition (PCM) is extremely frequent in hospitalized patients (Bistrian, Blackburn, Vitale, Cochran, & Naylor, 1976). The frequency among subjects beyond the age of 65 has not been adequately documented. This age-group does constitute the majority of hospitalized patients and experiences the highest prevalence of malnutrition. It is becoming more common for elderly patients to be admitted to the hospital with PCM as their primary diagnosis; however, the malnutrition is usually secondary to another disease (Lipschitz, 1982). The diagnosis of PCM in the hospitalized elderly is often relatively difficult because many of the alterations that occur as a result of PCM also occur as a part of the aging process (Lipschitz & Mitchell, 1982). It is important to recognize severe PCM in the elderly because it is so easy to improve nutritional status by appropriate nutritional therapy (Lipschitz & Mitchell, 1982) and because of the major effect that poor nutrient intake has on the ability of the malnourished individual to respond to stress, heal wounds, or fight infection. The normal body defense mechanisms are severely compromised. All of this results in an increased hospital stay, increased morbidity, and a decreased chance of responding to treatments aimed at correcting the primary disorder.

14
Surgery and Aged Women: Indications and Contraindications

Claude E. Welch

Several years ago in a lovely park in Oslo, Norway, my wife and I were privileged to see the Vigeland sculptures. Hundreds of them made by this famous artist portrayed life with great sensitivity. I will describe only two of them. One portrayed youth and the other old age. They emblazen a truth that we oldsters fain would forget—that what is appropriate for one age is not necessarily so for the other. The eyes of the youths are focused on the horizon, muscles firm and tense, ready for the vigorous encounters of life, facing their trials with confidence. But for the women in old age, the spark is gone. Dim eyes are turned to the soil from which they had sprung. Shrunken breasts, pendulous abdomens, and feeble arms speak of a body as withered as the spirit, and their faces cry with the wish for rest and peace.

They speak to us saying "Dear physician: Life has been hard. We have done our duty. There is little more that we can accomplish. Can you bring us new life, new hope, or at least comfort us and ease our infirmities?"

This is the task of the physician and of the surgeon who can, to some extent at least, reprieve the sentence of imminent death or make the ills of life more tolerable for aged women. As Dunphy (1968) has stated,

> The tradition is ancient that the physician and surgeon must do everything they can to promote, not just the health, but the comfort and well-being of their patients. It is of little value to cure disease if the cure is worse than the disease itself. Nor does it profit the patient to have a palliative operation which only permits him to live longer without alleviating his suffering. (p. 369)

194

What the surgeons should do or not do is quite different from what is required for younger persons, since in old age life expectancy will be measured in terms of a few years or months rather than decades. Prophylactic surgery to prevent future ills becomes of much less importance. On the other hand, urgent relief from serious illness that, if unresolved, would fill the remaining life with pain or disability is essential. It is only by such maneuvers that gnarled fingers and withered limbs can resume their rightful place in a society that today believes longevity is less important than the quality of life.

What can the surgeon accomplish? Can he or she befriend aged women, or can he in his zeal expose them and society to even greater difficulties? What do such women want? What can society afford? These are questions not easily answered, but I will discuss them, avoiding too many technical details.

Let us first consider what the surgeon can do to help aged women. At the outset we should seek factual data. The definition of old age varies. Medicare benefits begin at 65. Authors have used any age from 60 to 80 as the dividing line. Unless otherwise specified, in this chapter any woman 80 years or over qualifies as aged. We know that the average life expectancy of a woman at age 80 is about six years and declines rapidly thereafter. Women are much more durable than men. There is evidence concerning the mortality of operations conducted after age 80 (Table 14.1). Several years ago I analyzed a consecutive personal series of operations on 100 patients over 80 years of age (Welch, 1969). From ages 80 to 84 the mortality was 3 percent, from 85 to 89 it was 9 percent, and from 90 years of age and over it was 25 percent. Thus patients in the ninth decade of life tolerated operations well. They are reasonably tough or they would not have lived as long as they have. Postoperative complications, however, are much more common than in the young, and when one occurs many others are apt to follow just as Oliver Wendell Holmes portrayed in his story of the one-horse shay. Recent improvements in anesthesia have made operations much safer, and as a result one-stage procedures that correct pathology in one swoop have superceded most two- or three-stage operations that were advised more commonly years ago (Donaldson & Welch, 1968). Elective operations likewise have become more common, according to studies by Linn (e.g., Linn, Linn, & Wallen, 1982).

To give some general perspective on the necessity of surgical

TABLE 14.1
Operations and Mortality—
Personal Series[a]

Age	Cases	Operations	Deaths	Mortality (%)
80–94	67	72	2	3
85–89	26	31	3	9
90+	7	8	2	25
Total	100	111	7	6.3

[a]Adapted from "Surgery in the Twilight Years" by C. E. Welch, 1969, *Bulletin, 23'
Congres Societe de Chirurgie* (Buenos Aires), *September,* pp. 302–396.

TABLE 14.2
Mortality by Operation[a]

	Cases	Deaths
Herniorrhaphy	22	0
Colon resection		
Cancer	18	1
Diverticulitis	8	0
Gastric resection		
Cancer	7	0
Ulcer	8	0
Gallbladder		
Cholecystectomy +		
common duct exploration	11	1
Cholecystectomy	1	0
Cholecystostomy	2	1
Resection of rectum for cancer	5	0
Obstruction, small intestine	8	2
Other operations	21	2

[a]Adapted from "Surgery in the Twilight Years" by C. E. Welch, 1969, *Bulletin, 23'
Congres Societe de Chirurgie* (Buenos Aires), *September,* pp. 302–396.

procedures in older women, some indication of the incidence of acute abdominal complaints and the outcome in such patients is provided by Fenyö (1982). He studied two series of elderly patients in Sweden. About two-thirds of them were women. The first group consisted of 726 patients over 70 years of age admitted to the hospital between 1960 and 1965 for acute abdominal complaints. The second included 1000 patients seen in 1977 and 1978. Of the patients in the first period, 28.5 percent had surgery and in the second, 34.4 percent. The death rates fell in the second period after all common operations. The overall death rate decreased from 14 to 11 percent; this fall was tempered by the fact there was a great increase in malignant disease seen in the later series and this elevated the mortality rate.

Indications for operations vary in old age from those in middle age because elective operations must be considered very carefully and emergency procedures are correspondingly more common. In old age emergency operations include those for fractured hips, strangulated hernia, the complications of gallstones, intestinal obstruction, peripheral emboli, and intra-abdominal vascular catastrophies such as ruptured aortic aneurysm or mesenteric thrombosis. Elective operations include those for cancer (particularly of the breast, the colon, and the uterus), inguinal hernia, urinary incontinence, prolapse of the rectum, cataract, aortic aneurysms, and diseases of peripheral arteries.

Additional operations that are justified in younger women are not indicated in old age except in unusual circumstances. Such procedures include cosmetic surgery, extensive reconstructive dental procedures (except removal of teeth), open heart surgery, renal transplantation, joint replacements unless the patient has severe pain, and cholecystectomy for asymptomatic gallstones. However, it must be stressed that chronological and physiological ages are not necessarily equivalent. In a person "younger than her years" the indications for operation in the aged are essentially the same as they are for younger women. For data on mortality following some of these operations, see Table 14.2.

We will now examine in detail a few of the more important diseases in old women that can be ameliorated or cured by surgical procedures. They are hernias, gallstones, malignant disease, appendicitis, prolapse and incontinence, peripheral vascular disease, aortic aneurysms, and diseases of the hip joint.

DISEASES OF THE HIP JOINT

Fractures of the neck of the femur occur with great frequency in old women. Osteoporosis is more common in women than men. There is evidence that continued ingestion of estrogens after the menopause will retard the process. However, once begun, it is difficult to correct. These thin bones are likely to fracture with minor trauma.

The modern treatment of fractured hips consists either of fixation of the head of the femur to the shaft by metal pins, or excision and replacement of the head of the femur with a metal prosthesis. As a result the patient is able to resume ambulation in a short period and is relieved of pain. Contrasted with the treatment by complete bed rest for weeks that was required a few decades ago, followed by the common sequelae of bed sores, pneumonia, and pulmonary emboli, it is obvious that the new techniques are a tremendous advance.

Another disease that now has become very common is degenerative disease of the hip joint. The cause is unknown. Eventually every movement of this joint becomes exceedingly painful and the victim is reduced to immobility or crutches. Now pain can be relieved dramatically by operation and mobility can be returned. The operation is complicated and orthopedic surgeons advise it only when pain is so severe that relief is necessary.

PERIPHERAL VASCULAR DISEASE

There are two very common degenerative vascular diseases that may require surgery. The first is arteriosclerosis of the arteries of the lower extremities. Years ago as these arteries gradually occluded, gangrene followed. The only recourse was amputation, sometimes of the toes, but very frequently above the knee. Now grafts of veins or synthetic material can be employed in many instances so that the loss of a lower extremity can be avoided. Relief of the severe pain that accompanies gangrene and retention of the ability to walk represent enormous gains. A bilateral leg amputee was a particularly pitiful person; she often would be unable to get out of or even turn in bed without assistance.

A second manifestation of peripheral vascular disease that is amenable to surgery is that of so-called little strokes due to blocking of the carotid arteries. This disease now can be detected easily and relieved by a very simple procedure. The artery is opened, the clot removed, and circulation restored. In this way major strokes with severe disability or death can be avoided.

These operations are examples of prophylactic procedures that must be carried out before the major complication of gangrene of the leg or severe stroke supervene.

Karmody and Leather (1979) have studied the results of vascular surgery in the aged. Thirty-one of their patients had carotid surgery with no mortality. Eighty-three patients were faced with the loss of a limb because of arteriosclerosis of the arteries of the leg. Only 11 of them required major amputations. It was possible to restore circulation in 72 so that the maximum tissue loss was a portion of the foot.

MALIGNANT DISEASE

The older a woman becomes the more likely she is to develop cancer. There is no evidence to support the statement that cancer is less likely to pursue a fatal course in the old than in the young. Excluding cancer of the skin, which can be diagnosed early and treated effectively, the two most common manifestations in the older women are cancer of the breast and cancer of the large intestine.

Cancer of the breast should be diagnosed more easily in the old than in the young because of atrophy of normal breast tissue; however, older patients do not report to physicians as soon as they should. Operations usually are tolerated as well as they are in the young. Surgery should be prompt and adequate (Hunt, Fry, & Bland, 1980). Older women tolerate heavy doses of adjuvant therapy such as x-ray or chemotherapy poorly. Actually, chemotherapy is of doubtful value in the aged. Hormonal manipulation, on the other hand, may secure excellent palliation.

Cancer of the large intestine is the commonest form of internal cancer in old women. It also occurs more frequently on the right side where the symptoms of gross bleeding and change in bowel habits are not likely to occur. Unexplained anemia and symptoms of indigestion are typical. Fortunately, if detected at an early stage, the great majority of these patients can be cured by operation.

APPENDICITIS

Appendicitis is less common now in all age-groups than it was a few decades ago. In old age symptoms are apt to be atypical. For many years it has been the custom of many surgeons to remove the appendix at the time of some other abdominal operation since appendectomy under these circumstances is easy and will prevent any future attacks.

There is very little information concerning the frequency of appendicitis or appendectomy in any age-group. However, some interesting data were provided recently in the State of Wisconsin, where the number of these operations now is known. Investigators estimate that 1000 appendixes would need to be removed prophylactically to prevent one operation for appendicitis in the over-65 population (Nockerts, Detmer, & Fryback, 1980). Hence, on the assumption that these figures will be confirmed by others, this appears to be one operation to prevent future disease that previously was believed to be valuable but should be discredited.

HERNIA

This discussion will be limited to hernias that appear in the groin. There are several types but only two are common in old women. The most serious is femoral since it is often associated with strangulation and gangrene of the intestine. The other type—indirect inguinal—is less likely to strangulate but still is dangerous.

Tingwald and Cooperman (1982) studied the mortality and morbidity after inguinal and femoral hernia repairs in geriatric patients. For elective repair in 44 patients there were 8 postoperative complications but no deaths. For emergency repair in 18 cases there were 10 complications and 3 deaths.

Since emergency operations for strangulated hernia in the aged carry a high mortality, elective repair is advisable before strangulation occurs. The operation usually can be done under local anesthesia with minimum mortality.

AORTIC ANEURYSMS

Abdominal aortic aneurysms occur because of arteriosclerosis. They become more common as age advances. They are subject to rupture and can cause sudden death. As a result elective resection is advised for good-risk patients even in the aged. O'Donnell, Darling, and Linton (1976) found that the mortality of elective aneurysmectomy in patients over 80 was only 2 percent despite the fact that many had significant heart disease. Petracek, Lawson, Rhea, Ritchie, and Dean (1980) found that the mortality for resection of abdominal aneurysms in patients over 80 was similar to that for young persons. Their death rates were as follows: resection of 19 asymptomatic aneurysms was followed by 1 death (5.2%), 7 symptomatic aneurysms by 2 deaths (26.6%), and of 12 aneurysms with free rupture by 8 deaths (66.7%). Treiman et al. (1982) had a mortality rate of 8.6 percent for elective resections; 14 percent of the patients were alive 5 years later. Prophylactic resection of aneurysms 6 cm or more in diameter now is considered wise by most surgeons, assuming that there are no other serious contraindications.

GALLSTONES

Gallstones are extremely common, particularly in aged patients. Approximately a third of all autopsies done on persons over 70 will show gallstones.

Several reasons have been advanced for the removal of gallbladders that contain stones. Obviously when they cause pain or lead to severe inflammation, they should be removed. It has been estimated that about one out of 10 patients over 70 with acute inflammation of the gallbladder also have cancer of the gallbladder. It has also been found that old patients who have operations for stones in the gallbladder have them in many instances in the common duct as well. Stones in the common duct are particularly dangerous because they can lead to infection in the liver or pancreas.

Two reasons have been given for the removal of gallbladders that contain asymptomatic stones. The first is that given a long enough period of time, they are certain to become symptomatic. The other is that cancer tends to develop in gallbladders that contain stones. These arguments actually do not carry much weight in women over 80, and it is uncommon for elective cholecystectomy to be advised in women of that age provided they have not had any symptoms from their stones. On the other hand, if the stones have been symptomatic, then it will be preferable to remove the gallbladder at an elective time.

Sullivan, Hood, and Griffen (1982) had no deaths in 10 patients over 80 who had elective cholecystectomy. Of 32 patients operated on as emergencies, 4 died. Thirty-one percent of the patients had stones in the common duct as well as in the gallbladder.

PROLAPSE AND INCONTINENCE

Prolapse of either the uterus or the rectum can be a painful disease. Urinary and fecal incontinence often accompany prolapse but also may occur in the absence of any other lesions. These symptoms are particularly distressing because personal hygiene is difficult to maintain. Even old women, despite the fact that they are feeble and relatively poor risks, may require surgery for symptomatic relief. Though such operations may not be completely successful, they serve to ameliorate the troublesome symptoms.

CONTRAINDICATIONS TO SURGERY

The contraindications to operative procedures in the aged include those that are present in other groups. Some contraindications in patients of all ages can be righted by proper preoperative care. Severe anemia can be relieved by transfusions and total parenteral nutrition. A recent coronary thrombosis is a contraindication and it is necessary to wait several months before an operation can be carried out. Dementia and severe depression are much more serious problems in the aged because psychoses often are irreversible in the comparatively short span of life that is left. Consultation with psychiatrists in cooperation with the family is essential.

Some contraindications that are much more controversial deal with the social milieu in which the patient lives and is treated. Thus nursing home patients who are disoriented or severely handicapped and those whose status will be changed little by operation are not candidates for surgery. Other procedures that promise to have little return insofar as extension of life or improvement of quality of life must be instituted with caution. It is particularly in these cases that the overenthusiastic surgeon can be a foe to the patient and to the family. The utmost judgment and cooperation of all who are involved is essential. Too trivial an operation may be a useless exercise; too extensive an operation may be followed by a series of complications. The aim of the surgeon should be to help the patient but first to do no harm.

CONCERNS OF THE PATIENT

Since we have considered what the surgeon can accomplish, the next question is What do aged women desire? The surgeon must remember that many of them are depressed and the comfort and good cheer that he or she can offer can be as important as the operation. Alfred Worcester said

> The aged, as we must never forget, are always lonesome. They have outlived the preceding, and, very likely also their own generation . . . To the ways and manners of the present they are not accustomed. They belong to the unforgiving past. They are as strangers in the land. (Worcester, 1968, p. 348)

What faculties are important for aged women? Let me list the major ones. They wish to be independent, to think clearly, to see, to hear, to eat, and to excrete normally. They should be mobile, not confined to a bed, and preferably not to a wheelchair. They wish to be free of pain. They should be continent of urine and feces. As noted before, the surgeon can aid in the attainment of several of these desires. Prophylactic carotid surgery for transient ischemic attacks may prevent strokes. Removal of cataracts may restore sight. Surgical relief of arterial obstruction in legs and prompt nailing of fractured hips can maintain or restore mobility. At times incontinence can be relieved.

But not too much can be expected of the surgeon. He or she cannot restore the original healthy member or organ. There may be a price to pay—loss of a few toes for continued ambulation and a viable leg, or in very serious cases of fecal incontinence an abdominal stoma in exchange for an incompetent anus. Nor can the surgeon restore the élan and sparkle that distinguish good health from freedom from pain or disease. As Wilder Penfield wrote of old age:

> Toward the end, senescence with its comforting drowsiness closes stealthily one door after another. And so when death does come at last, it may not be unwelcome after all. (1968, p. 343)

Finally, let us turn to some of the severe ethical dilemmas that are forced upon the surgeon in the case of aged patients. There are two that seem to be of overriding importance, namely, the conflict between preservation of life and quality of life and the economic consequences of care of the aged.

It frequently is assumed that the physician should be dedicated to the preservation of life regardless of all other considerations. To do otherwise could lead by gradual transition to the evils that were portrayed in the Nuremberg trials and allow the physician to be an arbiter of life and death. In many respects, however, this is a modern problem; physicians who knew their individual patients a century ago were concerned chiefly with advice and comfort measures; pneumonia (the old folks' friend) would run its course unchecked in the aged. Today the enormous impersonal facilities provided by anesthesia, antibiotics, and the like make it more difficult for the physician to withhold treatment that in terminal cases may serve only to prolong suffering. Nursing homes usually return patients to hospitals when serious complications occur. When such ill patients are admitted to the hospital with many doctors in attendance, none of whom know the patient or family, it is difficult to restrain the system that aims to provide all the machinery of modern medicine to prolong the life of a dying patient. Lawyers, judges, and committees have combined to make it difficult and painful for the patient to die. On the other hand, "right to die" groups have urged that it is an individual right for a patient who is mentally competent, with the agreement of the family and the physician, to refuse extraordinary measures to prolong life.

The second dilemma concerns the economic costs of care of the aged. Statistics gathered by the government concerning payments made by Medicare show the great expenses involved in the hospital care of these patients. Furthermore, a high percentage of them die either in the hospital or within a year after discharge. In these days of stringent economic restrictions and excessive costs of hospitalization, pressures will almost surely rise to emphasize the value of an individual to society rather than to concentrate upon the preservation or even the quality of life.

Some statistics are of interest. According to data collected by the Massachusetts Health Council, from 1970 to 1980 the number of people over 85 increased by 48 percent in the United States. A person over 75 years of age used as many hospital days as eight younger adults. The health care costs for an oldster in Boston in

1980 was $3996. The annual costs of Medicare in the United States are over $20 billion, and life expectancy after hospitalization of a Medicare patient is low.

Is it just or moral to establish an age limit above which certain operations should not be performed? In England, for example, renal transplants are not allowed after the age of 60. Patients above this age who have cancer are given lower priorities on the waiting list. Of course, the aged are not as likely to clamor for an operation as younger persons, but is it fair to establish age as the sole criterion? It is perfectly clear that chronological age is not equivalent with physiological or anatomic age. Some people are burned out at age 50; others are competent and extremely effective up until age 90. Unfortunately, no one yet has been able to devise a system of measurement that would take these features into account, and so chronological age regardless of its deficiencies has remained an effective barrier. Certainly it is urgent that some change from the chronological age criterion should be considered and some better method be devised than the totally immoral restriction of benefits for certain patients after the age of 60.

The lack of economic return implies to economists that there is little point in offering older patients surgical relief of their disease and that the hospital and professional expenses that are incurred by these patients essentially result in a total economic loss for the country. It should be recognized, however, that operations in this age-group are not performed very frequently and comprise only about 1 percent of all the operations done. It would seem that our affluent society should be able to spend that much in the interest of compassion and comfort.

Ultimately the values bestowed by the surgeon must be evaluated by the results he or she has obtained. In the study referred to previously, I inquired from many families and patients as to whether or not they considered the operation worthwhile. In most instances the family, as well as the patient, was grateful for survival and extension of a more comfortable life. In nearly all cases the operation was an incident that did not change the usual pattern of life of the patient. Those patients who were productive prior to operation usually continued to be. It was uncommon for an operation to change a gainfully occupied person to an invalid or on the other hand to make a worker out of one who had been unemployed. In a few cases the patient became worse after operation, but in general these were the cases in which irreversible malignant disease was found. In some a successful operation was followed by hostility from the family and a retrospective statement that they wished the operation never had been done. Psychological factors are complex, but the surgeon may expect a transfer of a hostile reaction by the families of some patients in case the patient who is disliked by her relatives survived.

Many aged women make delightful patients. Witness the lady who told me after a serious operation not to tell her daughter, who thought her age was 83, that it actually was 89. Witness the lady of over 100 who read her poetry to me before and after another difficult operative procedure (Welch & Whittemore, 1954). When I asked her whether or not she had ever had a secretary, she said, "No, but I always wanted to have had an amanuensis." Consider another lady who postoperatively became a gold star mother and traveled abroad at age 90.

Thus surgeons can be either friends or foes to the patient and to society. They usually are friends when they extend a happy life span or carry out procedures that improve the quality of life and make it more tolerable. They can be foes if they advocate operations that convey questionable benefits or above all if what they do serves merely to prolong an uncomfortable, miserable existence. However, it must be said that the ethical problems have not been resolved to everyone's satisfaction. There are many who believe the sole duty of a physician should be to prolong life and therefore every attempt should be made to reverse a situation that is bound to be hopeless without surgery. There are some who believe that the economic drain posed by the care of older patients is so great that some alteration must be made. My personal sympathies obviously rest with those surgeons who would introduce compassion and care for the patient with preservation of quality rather than length of life and with the members of the public who believe that older women deserve this care regardless of the cost.

15
The Uses and Misuses of Pharmacology

CHARLES L. HOPPEL

INTRODUCTION

It is generally acknowledged that elderly patients have a different response to drugs than younger patients. Much of the information basis to support this has been anecdotal, at best. In the past few years, emphasis has been directed toward providing a sound scientific knowledge base to develop a rational approach to the use of drugs in a geriatric patient. These studies are obviously difficult because we do not have an adequate assessment of biological versus chronological age. Also, studies are confounded by the presence of disease and the role of environmental factors. Nevertheless, a pharmacological data base is being developed that, in part, amplifies and correlates with the known physiological changes occurring during aging. The purpose of this chapter is to briefly review those principles and concepts of clinical pharmacology that provide a rational approach to drug therapy. Because of the scope, for the most part primary references will not be given for each point but review articles will be used. Therefore, the reader may track down specific issues by using these review articles as the entry point.

The geriatric population represents about 11 to 12% of the total United States population, whereas they account for between 25 and 30% of the expenditures for prescription drugs. If over-the-counter drugs are added to this, the percentage would probably

Acknowledgment: The author would like to thank Dr. Lee-Ann Gilmer for reviewing the manuscript.

be even more impressive. The elderly have more chronic illnesses and multiple medical problems. They, therefore, have indications for multiple drugs and, with polypharmacy, they are subject to and experience more adverse drug reactions.

The fundamental pharmacological principles needed to understand the therapeutic dilemma and some of the reasons for the increased incidence of adverse reactions can be considered under two headings.

1. Pharmacokinetics: The time course whereby the drug gets to its site of action. This includes absorption, distribution and elimination of the drug.

We will discuss the known effects of aging on these processes and possible implication from multiple drug therapy.

2. Pharmacodynamics: The relationship between the drug at its site of action and the receptor for the action of the drug.

Either of these two basic concepts can provide a mechanism for an exaggerated or decreased effect and an adverse effect.

It is important to emphasize that a necessary foundation (Hollister, 1981; Ouslander, 1981) must be laid for proper drug therapy that includes:

1. A proper diagnosis;
2. A decision that pharmacological treatment is necessary;
3. Clearly defined objectives;
4. An informed patient and/or family unit;
5. A decision that as few drugs as possible will be administered as simply as possible; and
6. An understanding that therapy will be assessed taking compliance into consideration.

Common sense must be exercised; for example, if the patient cannot read the label on the medication because the print is too small, he or she may rely on a less than perfect recollection of instructions and inappropriately take the medication. The fewest number of essential drugs and administration by the simplest regimen are highly desirable.

PHARMACOKINETICS

Pharmacokinetic mechanisms may play a role in determining an individual's response to a drug. They describe the time course for the appearance, distribution, and disappearance of a drug in the body. The absorption, distribution, protein-binding, and elimination of a drug are included in determining the onset of action and duration of action of a drug. A few concepts are necessary to appreciate these pharmacokinetics.

If we administer a drug by an intravenous route, the total dose given is delivered to the systemic circulation. The drug can then diffuse out of the circulation into extracellular fluid or other compartments, such as tissues. The drug can also be eliminated by either metabolism (usually the liver) or excretion (usually the kidneys). If we think of the body as a tub of water and we add a known amount of drug to that tub and it is mixed, the concentration of drug in the water will enable us to determine how much water is in the tub.

$$\text{Concentration} = \frac{\text{Amount added}}{\text{Volume}}$$

therefore

$$\text{Volume} = \frac{\text{Amount added}}{\text{Concentration}}$$

This same concept is used to express the volume of distribution of drug in the body. Although we could approach drug distribution mathematically, as a simple concept, we can look at a drug after it has been distributed, and *assuming* that the concentration outside the systemic circulation is the same as the plasma concentration, from measurement of plasma concentrations and the amount injected intravenously we can calculate volume of distribution (V_D) as we did above for the tub of water. It is obvious that this term, V_D, is not defining an anatomical space but is treating the whole body as if it were similar to plasma. A drug with a small V_D would suggest that the drug is primarily distributed in the plasma compartment, whereas a large V_D would imply that the drug is sequestered in tissues.

The rate of removal of most drugs from the body is directly proportional to the concentration of the drug. This describes a first-order process. Therefore, if we plot the plasma concentration of a drug versus time using semilogarithmic paper, the plot will be linear. From this we can determine the time necessary for the plasma concentration to decrease 50 percent or the half-life ($t_{1/2}$). The half-life will be the same whether the drug decreases from 10 mg/ liter plasma to 5 mg/liter or from 5 mg/liter to 2.5 mg/liter. The elimination constant (β) can be determined, which is the slope of this linear decay. The half-life and the elimination constant of the first-order process are related by the following:

$$t_{1/2} = \frac{\ln (2)}{\beta} = \frac{0.693}{\beta}$$

These are important factors in describing the elimination of a drug from the body.

The most important determination for describing the elimination of a drug is its clearance. Clearance of a drug is described, just like clearance in a physiological sense, as the volume of plasma completely cleared of the drug per unit of time. Clearance (Cl) is related to the volume of distribution and the elimination constant (or $t_{1/2}$):

$$Cl = V_D \cdot \beta = \frac{0.693 V_D}{t_{1/2}}$$

by substituting $t_{1/2}$ for β using the above definition. The plasma clearance does not provide an answer to how or where the drug is cleared. It is the sum of the renal clearance and metabolic (usually hepatic) clearance of the drug. Obviously, these components vary depending on the drug being discussed.

A last and very important pharmacokinetic concept is the attainment of a steady-state plasma concentration. At steady state, the amount of drug that gets into the body will be the same as the amount that is eliminated. This occurs when we regularly take a drug over time. Therefore, we know the dose ingested, how often it is taken, and the bioavailability of that drug. Bioavailability is defined as the percentage of the ingested dose that enters the systemic circulation. For a drug given intravenously it will be 100 percent, whereas for orally administered drugs the bioavailability is dependent on the drug itself and the form in which it is taken, e.g., type of tablet.

Clearance describes the elimination. Therefore, at steady state the plasma concentration (C_{SS}) of a drug is given by the following relationship:

$$C_{SS} = \frac{\text{Dose per dosing interval}}{\text{Clearance}}$$

If the drug is not completely bioavailable, then the dose integrated will have to be adjusted to reflect the amount actually entering the systemic circulation.

From the relationship for steady-state plasma concentration, it is clear, assuming no changes in dosing of a drug, that clearance is the critical factor in determining the concentration. There are wide interindividual differences in the clearance of a drug, with the consequence that doses of drugs must be individualized. We will examine the effect of aging on clearance and the factors that comprise clearance. Furthermore, with multiple drug therapy, the influence of one drug on the clearance of another drug is a major factor in determining drug interactions.

The monitoring of the plasma concentration of drugs to ascertain the actual amount of drug in the body is clearly superior to the use of the dose administered. Two individuals may require markedly different doses to attain the same steady-state plasma concentration. Inherent in this discussion is the idea that the plasma concentration reflects the concentration of drug at its site of action and thus the pharmacological or toxic effect.

Absorption

Physiological changes that occur in the gastrointestinal tract with aging have been described (Greenblatt, Sellers, & Shader, 1982; Hollister, 1982; Lamy, 1982; Ouslander, 1981; Vestal, 1982). These include a decrease in the gastric parietal cell function leading to a decrease in gastric acid secretion and thus an increase in gastric pH. The motility of the gastrointestinal tract is less in the elderly, and gastric emptying is slowed. The absorptive surface has been described as being decreased. Furthermore, the splanchnic blood flow is decreased. Some nutrients that are absorbed by active transport have been shown to have impaired uptake in the gastrointestinal tract. In contrast, drug absorption in the elderly is not grossly decreased, either in rate or in extent of absorption. A slight delay in the absorption of digoxin and chlordiazepoxide has been reported. Why is there this essentially unaltered absorption of drugs in the elderly in the face of the known physiological changes? Most drugs are absorbed by passive non-ionic diffusion, principally in the small intestine, and this process would not be expected to be markedly influenced by the known alterations.

Distribution

The distribution of drugs may be influenced by the changes in body composition that occurs with aging (Greenblatt et al., 1982; Hollister, 1982; Lamy, 1982; Ouslander, 1981; Vestal, 1982). Total body water decreases with age with decreases in plasma and extracellular volume. In women, there is a decrease in lean body mass, whereas there is an increase from 33 to 48 percent in adipose tissue. Therefore, drugs that are relatively soluble in water and that are distributed in body water or lean body mass would be expected to have altered volumes of distribution. Such drugs as acetaminophen or digoxin have been shown to have decreased volumes of distribution. On the other hand, because of the larger percent of body fat, drugs that are more lipid-soluble may be predicted to have larger volumes of distribution. A significant increase in the distribution of diazepam, a benzodiazepine, has been noted.

Since women have a greater percentage of body fat and less lean body mass, this would be expected to further compound the age-related changes in distribution. In fact, the distribution of diazepam (highly lipid-soluble) is more extensive in women and conversely the distribution of acetaminophen (water-soluble) is decreased.

With age the cardiac output decreases as does blood flow to the liver and kidneys. These changes result in about a 40 to 45 percent reduction in liver blood flow (Geokas & Haverback, 1969).

Another factor that can influence the distribution of drugs is protein-binding. Plasma albumin concentrations decrease with age, and illness or poor nutrition can cause further significant declines (Greenblatt, 1979; MacLennan, Martin, & Mason, 1977;

Wallace & Whiting, 1976). The reduction in plasma albumin will provide fewer binding sites in plasma for drugs that are highly bound to albumin. Therefore, at a particular total plasma concentration of a drug that is highly bound to albumin, the percentage of free drug will be increased, as will the concentration of free drug relative to the situation where plasma albumin is normal. It is free drug in plasma that is in equilibrium with the distribution space and with the concentration of drug at the active site and at sites of elimination. Because we measure total drug concentration in most instances of therapeutic drug monitoring, these changes in plasma albumin will influence the interpretation of the plasma concentration versus pharmacological effect. The therapeutic change for total drug in plasma would be expected to be shifted toward lower values because of the increase in free fraction. The measurement of plasma free drug concentrations would provide the best estimate of the drug at its site of action.

Phenytoin, salicylate, warfarin, and tolbutamine have decreased protein binding in the older aged subject. Polypharmacy complicates the problem for highly bound drugs and competition for binding sites may further increase the free fraction.

Elimination

The elimination of drugs from the plasma compartment and body occurs primarily by two routes: (1) metabolism in the liver; and (2) excretion by the kidney (Greenblatt et al., 1982; Hollister, 1982; Lamy, 1982; Ouslander, 1981; Vestal, 1982). The clearance of drug from the plasma will be dependent on these two processes, although biliary excretion does play a minor role.

Hepatic Metabolism. The metabolism of a drug in the liver, in general, produces a more water-soluble derivative. The metabolite may be inactive or active from a pharmacological standpoint, which may be a significant factor in the aged as opposed to the young. Liver weight decreases with age as does the blood flow. Antipyrine is an agent that is frequently used to measure oxidative metabolism. The metabolic clearance of antipyrine is decreased in the elderly and is more pronounced in smokers than in nonsmokers; age may play only a minor role (Vestal et al., 1975). There is some evidence that the decrease in clearance of some drugs (e.g., antipyrine and diazepam) is greater in aging men than in women. The changes in oxidative metabolism associated with aging are drug specific but can lead to significantly lowered drug clearance and, thus, to higher plasma concentrations at steady state. The conjugation reactions do not seem to be greatly affected by aging. Additionally, the acetylation of drugs is not affected by aging.

The genetically determined fast and slow acetylators are found in the elderly without a change in the proportion.

The change in liver blood flow would be expected to alter the kinetics of drugs whose clearance is dependent on liver blood flow. The clearance of propanolol and indocyanine green are delayed in the elderly. In contrast, lidocaine clearance is not affected by age, although the volume of distribution is larger and the half-life is longer (Nation, Triggs, & Selig, 1976). Therefore, liver blood flow decreases with age, but the significance of changes in the intrinsic clearance (measure of the ability to remove drug by metabolism or biliary excretion) is dependent on the specific drug. Other factors, such as smoking, may have less effect in the aging.

Renal Excretion. The glomerular filtration rate and tubular excretory capacity decrease with aging. This is due to a decrease in renal blood flow and a decrease in nephrons. The decline is glomerular filtration rate averages about 35 percent. Therefore, drugs that are eliminated primarily by renal clearance would be expected to show a decline in clearance. To account for the decline in renal function, the creatinine clearance will adequately estimate glomerular filtration rate. Serum creatinine cannot be used as an index since muscle mass decreases with age and, therefore, endogenous creatinine production is likewise reduced. The production rate and clearance decreases together result in an unchanged serum creatinine. The creatinine clearance would have to decrease markedly to produce an increase in serum creatinine.

Drugs sugh as digoxin, cimetidine, chlorpropamide, and antimicrobials (aminoglycosides and penicillins) show reduced clearance in aging. Procainamide and its active metabolite, acetylprocainamide, are cleared by the kidney and show the expected decrease in clearance with aging.

PHARMACODYNAMICS

The development of toxicity at the usual therapeutic dose in the elderly led to the notion that receptor sensitivity was increased (Greenblatt et al., 1982; Lamy, 1982; Ouslander, 1981; Vestal, 1982). The impaired renal and hepatic function may explain most of the observed changes. An increase in sensitivity to the barbiturates seems accepted in the elderly. Impaired metabolism and renal excretion may be partly responsible for this effect.

The benzodiazepines have been carefully studied and the elderly seem to be more sensitive to diazepam and nitrazepam when plasma concentrations are equivalent. These data support the concept that the central nervous system is more sensitive to these benzodiazepines.

Older individuals seem to be more resistant to the cardiac effects of either beta-agonists (isoproterenol) or beta-antagonists (propanolol) (Vestal, Wood, & Shand, 1979). The mechanism for this alteration is not known but postreceptor changes are proposed.

Age also seems to be a determinant in the sensitivity to warfarin, which does not appear to be caused by pharmacokinetic factors (Shepherd, Hewick, Moreland, & Stevenson, 1977). An increased incidence of bleeding in women over 60 taking heparin has been noted (Jick, Slone, Borda, & Shapiro, 1968). It may reflect an increased sensitivity to heparin in the elderly women compared to young women and to men. There are no pharmacokinetic data on heparin to evaluate this aspect in the elderly.

ADVERSE DRUG REACTIONS

The incidence of adverse drug reactions in patients is much higher in the elderly (Hurwitz, 1969; Seidel, Thorton, Smith, & Cluff, 1966). The pharmacokinetic, pharmacodynamic, biochemical, and physiological factors that may play a role in this increased incidence have been discussed above under the appropriate subheading. Drugs are one of the most common causes of sudden, unexplained mental impairment in the older adult. For example, one study found that 16 percent of 236 patients over 65 years old were hospitalized for behavioral disturbances directly attributable to drugs (Learoyd, 1972). This is not surprising since there is a selective decline in some of the central nervous system pathways and preservation of others.

SUMMARY

How pharmacokinetics and pharmacodynamics differ in the aged is dependent on both the characteristics of the patient and the drug. There does not appear to be a marked alteration in the absorption of drugs in the elderly. In contrast, the decrease in lean body mass and total body water with an increased amount of body fat influences the distribution of drugs. In general in the elderly women, there is a decreased volume of distribution for the more water-soluble drugs, whereas there is an increased volume of distribution for the lipid-soluble drugs.

The clearance of drugs is the most important kinetic determination of drug handling by the body. The hepatic clearance of drugs, in the elderly, is influenced by the decrease in liver blood flow and the decrease in metabolic activity for some but not all drugs. Renal clearance of drugs is decreased by decreased renal blood flow, decreased glomerular filtration rate, and decreased tubular secretion.

Receptor sensitivity to drugs has been proposed to be altered in the elderly, but further studies are needed to address the mechanisms for these responses. Prospective studies are also needed to assess the qualitative and quantitative changes of drug handling in the elderly population. Furthermore, longitudinal studies are ultimately needed to assess the significance of the changes.

PART VI
HEALTH CARE ISSUES

Kahana and Kahana open this section with a thoughtful review of the literature on the effects of nursing home residence on elderly persons. They point out that the literature generally suffers from a lack of theoretical perspective and reports ambiguous or contradictory findings regarding the mortality, well-being, adjustment, and types of treatment outcomes. Their own research using a multivariate approach and three years of follow-up also raised more questions than it answered. Clearly the outcomes of institutionalization must still be unraveled, although these authors generally reject the view that institutionalization always has a negative outcome.

Next Vallbona and Baker present the effects on the functional capacity of aged persons of physical training and conditioning. The many benefits of exercise and movement on muscular, cardiac, and respiratory function are outlined. They close with a call for primary care professionals to use this information in counseling and treating aged persons. One might have wished for more application of this approach to persons who have suffered strokes or who are disabled with arthritis.

Many of the diseases experienced by aged women would have been prevented or at least lessened in their severity if a more healthful lifestyle had been practiced. In the final chapter in this section, Abdellah cites the national policy regarding maintaining the health of the citizenry and calls for early treatment as well as prevention programs in the community. She concludes with a list of research needed, as viewed from her perspective as the Deputy Surgeon General and Chief Nurse Officer of the U.S. Public Health Service. Of particular note are several topics not covered in this book, such as stress incontinence (a particularly vexing problem for the ambulatory and institutionalized older woman), treatable loss of vision and hearing, and the prevention, early detection, and treatment of all kinds of cancer.

The health care systems discussed in this section are limited to nursing homes, the rehabilitation setting, and, rather tangentially, the community. Three years ago an entire book sponsored by the Center on Aging and Health focused on the physician and the older patient. That aspect of the health care system was amply presented there. The "fit" between older women patients and the acute care hospital is also problematic. More aged women experience acute care hospitalization than experience nursing home care. Studies of the impact of this aspect of health delivery are clearly needed.

M. S.

16
Institutionalization of the Aged Woman: Bane or Blessing?

EVA KAHANA AND
BOAZ KAHANA

The impact of institutional living on older women represents an important but thus far largely neglected concern for social gerontologists. One obvious reason for focusing on the effects of institutionalization on the older woman is that the vast majority of institutionalized persons happen to be women. The National Nursing Home Survey (Van Nostrand, 1981) depicts the institutionalized person as:

> female, widowed, white, age 81, who has a disease of the circulatory system as a primary diagnosis, and who depends on assistance to bathe, dress, use the bathroom and get about. (p. 403)

According to the 1970 census data there were approximately 650,000 females over 65 residing in institutions (U.S. Department of Commerce, 1973). It has been estimated that an individual's chances of eventually living in a nursing home are about one in four (Palmore, 1976).

Furthermore, it has often been argued that age and female sex represent double jeopardies. Does institutionalization add to these disadvantages resulting in triple jeopardy? Elderly men and women experience different patterns of socialization, fulfill different social roles throughout life, and show different adaptations to the aging process (Beeson, 1975; Payne & Whittington, 1976; Rosen & Neugarten, 1964). Consequently, it is important to consider whether institutional living presents special problems for or poses special opportunities to older women.

In addition to the specific concern dealing with special characteristics, needs, and adaptations of older women, a more general question is also implicit in our topic. Is institutionalization in fact the end of the road, a bleak and dehumanized living arrangement for those older persons who cannot or will not be cared for by their families or community? Or is just the opposite the case, with life in institutions representing a legitimate alternative lifestyle or at the very least, professional care for those aged who can no longer live independently?

Although familiarity with the literature suggests several quick answers to these questions, upon closer scrutiny, the complexity of the issues quickly surfaces and one's conclusions may differ sharply depending on one's vantage point: the classical sociological literature, recent quantitative studies from the field of psychology, the sex roles literature, the clinical psychological literature, recent articles in applied gerontology, or views of nursing home administrators or consumer groups.

We will first address the most basic issue regarding the general impact of institutions: are they a bane or a blessing? Curiously, much of the institutional literature does not specifically deal with this question. The focus is instead on mediators of well-being among the institutionalized aged. Many of our conclusions have to be inferred from studies that do not consider whether residents fare well, but ask instead, "Who fares best and which environmental features promote adjustment in institutions?"

Although the vast majority of studies on institutional living are based on samples consisting predominantly or exclusively of older women, ironically there are few references in the gerontological literature to the special needs of older women in institutions. Among 37 recent studies of institutionalization considered for this review, only 9 (25%) *considered* sex differences and only 13% *reported* the existence of sex differences. In addition to summarizing results of relevant studies, findings will also be reported based on our own research regarding sex differences in institutional placement and in adaptation to institutional living.

DEHUMANIZING ASPECTS OF
INSTITUTIONAL LIVING

Analyses that have taken a holistic, qualitative view based on observations of institutional life at a close range depict the depersonalizing and dehumanizing effects of institutional living (Gubrium,

1975). From Goffman's (1961) descriptions of the total institution to Jules Henry's (1963) anthropological accounts of human obsolescence, their conclusions are unequivocal. The impact of the institution on residents is seen as devastating. In Henry's terms:

> In many primitive societies the soul is imagined to leave the body at death or just prior to it—here, on the other hand, society drives out the remnants of the soul of the institutionalized old person, while it struggles to keep his body alive. Routinization in attention, carelessness and deprivation of communications—the chance to talk, to respond, to read, to see pictures on the wall, to be called by one's name rather than "you," or no name at all—are ways in which millions of once useful but now obsolete human beings are detached from their selves long before they are lowered into the grave. (p. 393)

Exposés of the nursing home industry have ranged from Townsend's (1964) classic survey of life in British institutions to Mendelson's (1974) inventory of abuse and inequities in nursing home care in the United States.

The terms "institutional syndrome" (Tobin & Lieberman, 1976; Zusman, 1967) and "institutional neurosis" (Butler & Lewis, 1977) have been used to describe behavior of institutionalized older persons that is seen as reflecting apathy, lack of initiative, loss of interest, submissiveness, and resigned helplessness. Institutions have been charged with encouraging passivity in residents by overmedicating them, forcing them into a common mold, and treating them like dependent children (Gresham, 1976). Personal abuse of residents may result from untrained, unmotivated, and poorly supervised staff (Butler & Lewis, 1977).

For the aged person living in an institution, emphasis is usually on the most basic physical needs. It has been charged that even our better institutions for the aged operate on a "pathology model of aging," which views the individual as a medical management problem. As a result, the "sick" role may be readily adopted by the aged who enter institutional settings to live up to the expectations of illness (Coe, 1965). Even systematic observational studies of nursing homes yield data pointing to inactivity and lack of meaningful engagement (Gottesman & Bourestom, 1974). The extent to which staff of homes for the aged can look beyond disability, diminished function, and illness and see a *person* may be important in establishing the overall self-conceptions of the aged individual and may reflect the extent of therapeutic orientation in the home (E. Kahana, 1973).

DOES INSTITUTIONALIZATION LEAD
TO INCREASED MORTALITY?

One of the most alarming and readily understood ill effects cited for institutionalization has been that of increased mortality. Several studies have reported high death rates among new residents of institutions for the aged (reviewed in Rowland, 1977). The rates reported (i.e., 16–25% dead after one month) are considerably higher than those expected for the elderly in the general population.

In considering the possible negative effects of institutionalization, poor diet, infection, poor medical care, and sensory deprivation have been cited as factors that would be responsible for increased mortality rates (Butler & Lewis, 1977).

The dramatic conclusion based on these findings is typically that institutionalization hastens death. Nevertheless, the data lend themselves to alternative interpretations, the major one being that of selection bias. Thus, it is likely that older people enter institutions because of health problems and their health status is not comparable to that of the general population (M. A. Lieberman, 1969).

Findings based on a more refined methodology by use of a comparison group of aged on a waiting list to institutions and those institutionalized have generally confirmed conclusions that rate of deaths is higher among institutionalized than among waiting list elderly (M. A. Lieberman, 1969; Costello & Tanaka, 1961). These data have also been criticized, however (Kasl, 1972). The length of time on waiting lists and in institutions was not always strictly comparable and there may have been selective admission of the more frail and infirm from the waiting lists to the institution. A major problem inherent in these comparisons is the fact that experimental designs that would randomly assign persons to remain in the community or enter institutions are not feasible. Even if we were to establish conclusively that there is increased mortality subsequent to institutionalization, we would still be left with the question about attribution of those effects to relocation or to institutionalization *per se*.

More sophisticated statistical techniques are now being applied to addressing the issue of differential community and instituional mortality. In a recent article (McConnel & Deljavan, 1982), national level data were used from the National Nursing Home Survey of 1977 to measure differential nursing home and community death rates. Although the nursing home mortality rate is generally estimated to be 2 to 2½ times that of the age standardized community rate, the authors present evidence to demonstrate that adjusted for measurement errors the two rates are not in fact significantly different. (The differential was reduced from 156/1000 to 35/1000 and may be even less).

Sex Differences in Mortality

Among the many studies reviewed in considering differential institutional/community mortality rates, very few specifically addressed the issue of sex differences. Generally it is reported that men are more likely to die during the first year after entering a home for the aged (M. A. Lieberman, 1969). Goldfarb (1969) also found higher death rates among males entering three types of institutions. Higher mortality rates have also been reported for males who are transferred from one institution to another than for female patients (Pablo, 1977). Blenkner (1967) suggested that the minority status of males in institutions may contribute to their high death rate. In contrast, findings of a study by Bourestom and Pastalan (1972) revealed that among those elderly who died within a short period following institutionalization, the most vulnerable were the *older, female* most recently admitted individuals.

In considering these findings, one must of course take into account the generally higher mortality rate of males and possible selection factors operating.

POSITIVE ASPECTS OF INSTITUTIONAL LIVING

In striking contrast to the positions by critics of institutional care are the views of the advocates of institutional care. The consumer considering entry to an institution is typically provided information extolling the benefits of institutional living. Even from a scientific point of view, the potential positive impact of institutional living cannot be overlooked, especially when one considers environmental opportunities for previously isolated and impaired elderly. Positive outcomes are most likely to occur in high-quality facilities (Sherwood, 1975). Such institutions attest to the potential benefits of institutional living. Older persons whose social contacts in the community may be limited because of lack of transportation, lack of mobility, or health problems may find enhanced social opportunities. Proximity to persons of similar age and backgrounds has been found to result in expanded social interactions for some institutionalized elderly (Hendricks, Hetzel, & Kahana, 1978). Institutional living also provides opportunities for involvement in activities and social participation in a patient subculture. The activities surrounding the resident provide sources of stimulation as well. Studies by Tobin and Lieberman (1976) have also indicated considerable stability in self-conceptions among the elderly in the course of a year of institutional living.

Institutionalization can also result in marked improvements in diet, exercise, and medical care. Regularized nutrition in many cases corrects poor eating habits that older persons living alone may have slipped into. Older persons living alone often develop a pattern of self-neglect. They may be subsisting on tea, toast, and jelly, getting little exercise, and maintaining poor hygiene. Moving into a good institutional facility can serve to ameliorate such problems and improve their level of functioning. The availability of medical and nursing staff also provides a greater sense of security to both the older person and his or her family.

There is research evidence (Levey, Ruchlin, Stotsky, Kinlock, and Oppenheim, 1973) that quality of care in nursing homes has been considerably enhanced during the 1965–1969 time period. Efforts of consumer groups and increasing accountability have no doubt contributed to quality control in long-term care delivery (Anderson, 1974). Furthermore, there are indications from recent research (Kahana & Kiyak, 1982, 1983) that both staff attitudes and staff behaviors in diverse institutional facilities for the elderly are generally positive and facilitative of gratifying patient–staff interactions.

Institutionalization has often been viewed as reflecting the failure of the family support system. Yet recent empirical data do not support this view (Shanas & Maddox, 1976). Accordingly, Smith and Bengtson (1979) report that, in fact, institutionalization may often enhance family relationships between older persons and their adult children, i.e., negative changes occurred in only 10 percent of cases where postinstitutional family interactions were studied.

In a recent longitudinal study, Spasoff et al. (1978) reported that many older persons interviewed after entering an institution reported great relief after the move. One month after admission, most had made a satisfactory adjustment, although some were experiencing problems. Upon the six-month follow-up the vast majority reported good adjustment. Improvements in health were also reported, although these were tempered by increased dependency on staff. During a one-year follow-up, researchers report high levels of overall satisfaction, with 85 percent reporting that they are satisfied. In considering these results, we do need to keep in mind that reported satisfaction with institutional living may also be viewed as an index of acquiescence or of attempts to reduce cognitive dissonance and is seen by many as a questionable indicator of well-being (Carp, 1975).

Our own research has also pointed to generally benign influences of institutional living in a longitudinal study of 258 institutionalized older persons that we conducted in Michigan and Ohio (Kahana & Kahana, 1979). Results revealed no significant differences in health, morale, self-esteem, or mental status between time of admission and follow-up one year later.

Therapeutic programs of various forms conducted in institutional settings have also been demonstrated to enhance patient functioning (P. Beck, 1982; Dye & Erber, 1981; B. Kahana, 1975; Koger, 1980; Miller & LeLieuvre, 1982). Innovative programs have provided older persons with better coping skills (B. Kahana, 1975) and an enhanced control over their environment (P. Beck, 1982) with encouraging results. These findings generally demonstrate that older institutionalized persons can respond well to diverse psychological and social approaches directed at improving their level of functioning.

PREDICTION OF WELL-BEING
IN INSTITUTIONS

Research on the impact of institutional living on older persons in general, and older women in particular, typically focuses on predictions of diverse positive outcomes among persons who are institutionalized. Outcomes considered are generally morale, life satisfaction, and satisfaction with care or with the environment. Exogenous variables fall into three major categories. First are those studies that consider individual demographic or psychosocial characteristics as predictors of postinstitutional adjustment. The most popular predictors in recent research have been locus of control, social integration, conformity and attitudes toward diverse aspects of institutional life (B. Kahana, 1982). Accordingly, Schultz and Brenner (1977) and Langer and Rodin (1976) have found evidence that internal locus of control relates to greater psychological well-being among institutionalized aged. In contrast, Felton and Kahana (1974) observed more favorable outcomes among institutional residents who attributed locus of control to others. Instrumental and escape-oriented coping styles have also been found to correlate with higher morale among institutionalized elderly (Kahana & Kahana, 1979), as did assertive modes of adaptation (Tobin & Lieberman, 1976).

A second group of studies has focused on diverse environmental characteristics and features for their impact on resident adjustment. Organizational characteristics, such as institutional totality, privacy, institutional control, activities, and personal environments, e.g., resident rooms, have been considered in this category (Kart & Manard, 1974; Felton & Kahana, 1974). In particular, there is evidence of increased depersonalization and decreased morale among residents as a function of institutional size and totality (Lawton & Nahemow, 1973; Lowenthal & Robinson, 1976). Lack of physical privacy has been found to result in psychological withdrawal. Personalized environmental features in contrast have been found to contribute to enhanced interaction among nursing home residents (Lawton, 1970).

Last, a small group of studies has considered issues of person environment interaction such as areas of fit versus mismatch between environmental characteristics and personal preferences (Kahana, Liang, & Felton, 1980) as predictors of postinstitutional outcomes. M. A. Lieberman (1969) has argued that degree of discrepancy between pre- and postrelocation environment determines the amount of adaptation required of the older person who enters an institution. This genre of research aims to specify those conditions of both person and environment under which well-being of the institutionalized aged is maximized (Lawton & Nahemow, 1973).

METHODOLOGICAL ISSUES IN STUDIES
OF OLDER WOMEN IN INSTITUTIONS

In the social gerontological literature, there have been several approaches to the study of older women. First, there are large numbers of studies dealing with the aged that examine differences between older men and women. They follow the conventions, long accepted in the field, that gender makes a difference in individual characteristics, interaction patterns, personality dispositions, and even service needs. However, there is typically little concern in these studies with the special qualities, lifestyles, or experiences of women that would account for these sex differences. Second, there are numerous studies of the elderly that use older women for their sample. Older women are often chosen as study subjects simply because there are more of them or because they are more accessible. Thus we have studies of the effects of institutionalization in an "incidentally" female population. Last, there are the few investigations in very recent years that specifically focus on some aspect of life span development or deal with social issues from the perspective of the older woman. There have not been many studies directly addressing the issue of institutionalization focusing on older women.

The three trends referred to above are not, of course, mutually exclusive. Often the use of data and their interpretation are more critical in this context than is the nature of the data gathered. Furthermore, when studies focus only on women, omitting issues of sex differences, we are left with the critical question: Are the characteristics and relationships attributed to women in fact unique and do they differ from patterns that one would observe if groups of men had also been included in the study?

This is especially important in studies of aging and institutionalization where samples are often limited to women because of scarcity of older men, their unavailability, or their reluctance to participate in studies. Even studies that point out the existence of sex differences raise methodological problems. Such differences may in fact be due to special situations in which women find themselves but not be inherent in male–female differences (e.g., widowhood).

Sex differences in institutional adaptation may be expected based on differences in socialization of the two sexes. It has been generally argued that socialization of women has encouraged a more dependent and less assertive orientation than that of men (Payne & Whittington, 1976). However, in late life there is evidence that those norms have been transcended and more androgynous patterns of sex roles are manifested (Livson, 1976).

Much of what is known about sex differences in psychological development in late life is based on comparisons of middle-aged and/or young-old men and women (Neugarten & Guttmann, 1964). Such investigations indicate that as women age, they become more tolerant of their own aggressive and egocentric impulses. In contrast, men appear to become more tolerant of their nurturant and affiliative impulses. There is little information available, however, to indicate whether these trends persist in very late life and whether and how they are affected by institutionalization.

INSTITUTIONALIZATION OF OLDER WOMEN

Data available on institutionalization of older women may be roughly divided into two categories. First, there is information on sex differences in rates of institutionalization for older men and women. These differences have generally been attributed to differential social supports and differential service needs of the two sexes. Second, a relevant portion of the literature deals with adjustment and adaptation of elderly women or men within congregate or institutional facilities. Some information also exists on differences in treatment of men and women in institutional settings.

Entry to Institutions

The generalization that gets elaborated in many forms in the literature is that women have higher rates of institutionalization than men and that women overwhelmingly comprise the population of chronic care facilities. Three major reasons have been cited for differential rates of institutionalization for men and women:

1. The longer life expectancy of older women brings with it more chronic health problems that limit ability to function independently in the community.

2. The poorer economic situation of women precludes continued independent living when health problems arise.
3. Women tend to have less access to caretakers and more limited social supports, primarily because of widowhood.

Interestingly, the older the person is at the time of institutionalization, the more likely he or she is to have lived alone prior to admission. Conversely, the older the female patient, the less likely she is to be admitted from a hospital. At all ages men are more likely to be admitted to nursing homes from a hospital while women are more likely to be admitted from independent living arrangements (U.S. Department of Health, Education and Welfare, 1969). These data tend to support the contention that women are more likely to require institutionalization for social rather than medical reasons and hence, may be institutionalized in those situations when alternative community supports could permit more independent lifestyles.

In terms of social supports, older women are far more likely to lose their major social support, that is, their spouse, than are men. Their chances for remarriage are also diminished (Lopata, 1971). Research relating social support to service needs has clearly demonstrated that availability of a spouse is the single most important family support factor for reducing needs for formal services (E. Kahana, 1975). Data from a study on service needs of 300 elderly community residents in the Detroit area reveal older women living alone to be the most vulnerable group with limited resources and extensive immediate service needs (Kahana & Kiyak, 1980).

While the thrust of the research evidence points to a greater *social* vulnerability of the older woman, it is also important to note evidence to the contrary pointing out advantages she has regarding adjustment to life in institutions. Because of their expressive roles in the family, in old age women may find it easier to capitalize on already established kinship ties than men, who had seldom concentrated on maintaining kinship ties (Streib, 1975). These latter differences may lead us to expect that institutionalization of women would be delayed by assistance from family caretakers. It has been argued that men are more likely to turn to formal service providers after the death of their wives than are women after the death of their husbands. These arguments support stereotyped notions that older men, especially those living alone, are at a greater loss in managing tasks of household maintenance than older women because of their lack of experience or familiarity in performing household roles. Furthermore, women appear more concerned with their husband's health and anticipation of widowhood than with their own health or mortality (Neugarten, Wood, Kraines, & Loomis, 1963). In some cases a husband's frailty precipitates institutionalization for the wife as well. Concern for a husband's health and identification with the husband have been reported in some cases to hasten the dependent role for the older woman.

ADJUSTMENT OF WOMEN AND MEN IN INSTITUTIONS

When considering the relationship of sex and the effects of institutionalization a number of factors have to be considered. First, the nursing home is a female-centered institution (the majority of residents tend to be women), so behavioral norms may favor women. Second, as we have indicated, women and men may have different reasons for entering an institution. Third, health and mortality differ for the sexes, so women may live longer but tend to have more illness. Finally, male and female socialization differs. These differences were especially marked in the period around 1900 when the majority of persons who are currently institutionalized were born.

Women are generally seen as able to adapt more readily to institutional life than men. Nevertheless, there are many areas where women experience special problems, and there have been insufficient quantitative data to conclude that in fact women fare better.

While it may be useful to look at sex differences in adjustment, any major distinctions between men and women may relate to selection factors rather than being the result of institutionalization. Nevertheless, a survey of diverse studies does leave us with the suggestion that men and women may be affected in different ways by the experience of being institutionalized.

Lieberman and Lakin (1963) conducted a TAT study of elderly persons undergoing institutionalization. They suggest that for men the trauma of becoming institutionalized centers around a loss of self-worth or potency. The wish to be taken care of conflicts with the male's image as an independent and competent person. The major task here is reestablishment of a positive self-image after institutionalization. In contrast, for women, the basic problem in becoming institutionalized is a feeling of rejection by their children and by society at large. Their attempt at coping with this issue then is to establish themselves as "wanted" and well liked in the institution.

Transition from community to institutional life may thus be easier for females than for males because women experience less discontinuity in their social roles and fewer problems with becoming a dependent person. Yet related to their lifelong career as homemakers, institutionalization represents a particularly dramatic change in lifestyle of older women. In the institution they are greatly restricted in their ability to cook, clean, and care for the environment (Lieberman & Lakin, 1963).

In some sex role linked areas, women are likely to experience special frustrations upon being institutionalized. Giving up the role of homemaker may represent one such frustration to the older woman. In a study of conformity among institutionalized aged, Kahana and Coe (1969) found that elderly institutionalized women were particularly likely to show lack of conformity. Men were generally more able to observe food-related rules, whereas women had more difficulty in this area.

External locus of control has been found by Felton and Kahana (1974) to be more conducive to institutional adjustment than internal locus. In institutional settings where others are in fact in charge, attribution of locus of control to others may lead to less frustration. This may be one reason for easier adjustment by older women, who are more likely to exhibit external locus of control than do men (Palmore & Luikart, 1972). The patient role, which is a dependent one, assumes external locus on control and should be more familiar to women, who had lifelong patterns of dependency, than to men.

Women have been found more likely than men to be involved in planned and formal activities and to take leadership roles in congregate living environments. Men's social activity tended to be more casual and spontaneous (Zube, 1982). Women are more likely to express dissatisfaction, to complain, and to express feelings than men. Generally, greater help seeking by women has been documented both in medical sociology and gerontology literatures (Wolinsky, 1980). This does not necessarily indicate that in fact they are suffering from greater levels of illness, as suggested by their longer life expectancy.

There have been compelling presentations regarding the increased assertiveness, aggressiveness, and competence of the older or postparental woman (Rosen & Neugarten, 1964). Do these generalizations carry across to the aged women living in institutions?

In seeking to answer this question we must bear in mind that the institutionalized elderly represent the most vulnerable segment of the old-old group. Thus, we cannot assume that data about the psychological energy, strength, or aggressiveness of the young-old female persists through the many losses, jeopardies, and deprivations typically experienced by the older woman in her 80s who finds her way to an institution.

Accordingly, one must consider not only data on sex role differences between men and women but also differences in adaptation to illness as indicated by medical sociology literature. Pearlin and Schooler's work (1978) with stressful life events suggests that female socialization does not equip women to cope effectively with illness. Their traditional caregiver roles in the family may make acceptance of physical dependency more difficult. The notion of differential dependency of the sexes when it comes to assuming the sick role is a complex one. Men are generally discouraged in their socialization from acknowledging or communicating vulnerability, and are less likely to complain and seek help. Their adaptations tend to be more instrumental. The medical sociology literature acknowledges these paradoxes and points to "conceptually conflicting" contributions of sex to illness behavior (Lorber, 1981).

A few special problems noted for women in institutions deserve special attention. Bennett and Eisdorfer (1975) have argued that women may have special problems in adapting to congregate living since they have little or no school, camp, work, or army experience to help them adjust to regimentation.

A number of independent studies both in the United States and in Israel (Margulec, Librach, & Schadel, 1970) have indicated that women more frequently have accidents and falls in nursing homes than do male patients.

SEX DIFFERENCES IN TREATMENT

There is a good deal of anecdotal and clinical data that point to the fact women are treated differently from men by institutional staff. Staff are more reluctant to touch male than female patients

(Watson, 1975) and are likely to encourage and accept dependency on the part of older women. Nevertheless, it should also be noted that female patients often express discomfort at affective touching, especially by male attendants (DeWever, 1977).

Quantitative findings on sex differences in treatment relate primarily to the area of administration of drugs (Milleren, 1977). In long-term care facilities, females are more likely than males to receive major tranquilizers. Females are also more likely to be defined as anxious (more tranquilizers given even when level of anxiety is controlled for). Females also received higher doses of psychoactive drugs and were more frequently treated with several drugs than males in 12 U.S. hospitals.

Research dealing with sex differences in treatment of younger mental hospital patients (Doherty, 1978) generally points to more unfavorable treatment by staff of male than of female patients. Clinical observers have noted that at times men are treated with more respect than women, e.g., more likely to be called by their names. Yet there is also a harsher treatment of men for nonconformity because they are viewed as potentially more dangerous by staff than are older women.

RESULTS OF OUR RESEARCH
ON COPING WITH
INSTITUTIONALIZATION

Having reviewed evidence from research by others we now direct our attention to our longitudinal study of 287 persons who entered institutions and were followed for a three-year period, beginning prior to institutionalization (Kahana & Kahana, 1979). At the time of entry women outnumbered men 3 to 1 (there were 219 females and 68 males in the group admitted to 9 institutions). Interestingly, there were no significant differences in demographic or on selective factors in the two samples. The two groups had similar age distributions and previous living arrangements.

Men were significantly more likely to be married than women at entry. Thirty percent of the men who entered the homes were married compared to only 10 percent of the entering women. Men and women started out their institutional career portraying some interesting differences. Women had far better preparation for entry, typically making their own decisions to enter and coming from their homes. Men often entered from hospitals and felt that they did not make their own independent decision to enter the home. Women cited intergenerational reasons for entry, while men cited financial ones. Men reported significantly better health and portrayed higher morale on entry than did women. There were significant differences in coping styles, with women showing more affective and escape-oriented coping strategies, while men showed more instrumental coping styles (Kahana & Kahana, 1979).

Eight months after entry to the institution, men still reported better health than women, but differences in morale diminished over time with men and women showing more similar morale profiles. Women showed better social integration and more visits with other residents than did men.

Coping differences that existed prior to institutionalization did not shift to any appreciable degree. Women were still more likely to demonstrate escape and affective strategies as they did prior to entry into the home. It is noteworthy that affective strategies as opposed to instrumental ones were generally found to correlate with lower morale in our sample.

In summary, our own data do not lead us to conclude that women consistently fare better than men after institutionalization, as has been suggested in the literature. In certain areas females do better, while in others, males show more favorable reactions to institutionalization.

CONCLUSIONS AND FUTURE DIRECTIONS

Our review has revealed that generally literature has moved away from the bane or blessing concept of institutionalization to focus on intervening variables. Perhaps this reflects a greater appreciation of the complexities involved as compared to earlier approaches. Perhaps it is only begging the question. Even if we know that internal or external control enhances adjustment or which aspects of social integration are most beneficial, the question still remains. On the whole is institutionalization good for the aged woman or not?

The sociologists and anthropologists who have approached this question from a more phenomenological framework generally answer this question with a resounding conclusion: definitely a *bane*! On the other hand, as we have seen, a very different answer started emerging when a more unimpassioned, molecular, and multivariate approach was taken to this issue. Accordingly, more quantitatively oriented studies dissected out most of the malevolent influences suggested. Yet the recent quantitative studies are typically less in-depth and may miss the subjective experiences of dehumanization or depersonalization that have been attributed to institutional living.

Perhaps the answer to resolving these apparently contradictory positions lies in a recognition of the complexity of the phenomenon under study. In considering the institutionalized aged, one must realize that the variety of residential care settings is vast. Homes for the aged, nursing homes, chronic wards of general hospitals, and state mental institutions all serve elderly people with different types of problems. Furthermore, great variation exists in characteristics and quality of care provided by diverse facilities (Kosberg & Tobin, 1972). The impact of institutionalization must be considered in light of the special resources, limitations, and opportunities for alternative living arrangements that these aged possess.

We have few systematic guidelines about the most effective methods for maintaining high levels of psychosocial well-being. The far-reaching effects of behavior setting on participants have been well documented. Yet the psychological and social impact of behavior settings in which the elderly live is little understood at the present time. Understanding these environmental influences may point to possibilities for more effective therapeutic programs.

A humanistic approach to the treatment of institutionalized aged would suggest a less technical and more individual orientation in treatment programs. The striking absence of such programs in even many of the best of institutions may to a large extent be due to lack of a systematic theory of the psychosocial environment. What is very much needed, then, are environmental analyses that are relevant to the daily experiences of institutionalized older persons focusing separately on male and female patients.

How do the data on sex differences in institution adaptation stack up? In some sense they appear to favor the older woman. Yet it is also clear that different aspects of institutional life may be less problematic for men than for women. Ultimately, it may be far more useful to consider sex differences as important indices of the diversity of older patients than to look for sex as a major determinant of positive or negative institutional outcomes.

Perhaps this discussion does not leave one with a set of clear and simple conclusions about the special impact of institutionalization on the older woman. Nevertheless, we hope that it calls attention to the importance of considering the special characteristics and even diversity of older persons living in institutions.

Perhaps the lack of clear patterns is not altogether negative. We must come back to Dr. Riley's point (Chapter 1) regarding changing behavior norms, role expectations, and family structure and their impact on older women. Accordingly, the sex differences noted in the current research are likely to be transient and to represent part of an ongoing historical evolution.

17
Prospects for Rehabilitation of the Aged Woman

CARLOS VALLBONA AND
SUSAN BEGGS BAKER

A major challenge for health professionals in the decade of the 1980s is the establishment of coordinated multidisciplinary health programs for the elderly. Although the medical specialties that have become most involved in the development and implementation of such programs have been family medicine, internal medicine, physical medicine, and preventive medicine, specialists of numerous other disciplines are also becoming increasingly involved in the management of specific problems that occur very often in the geriatric population. Allied health professionals, especially nurses and social workers, have worked for many years in the care of the elderly. Their experience in home care and their observations in nursing homes have stimulated physicians to become interested in the health problems of the aged. The body of knowledge acquired by gerontologists in the last 20 years has provided the background and rationale for numerous research activities in the burgeoning field of geriatric medicine.

The prevention and the management of physical disability must receive particular attention in geriatric medicine because most elderly persons are not as physically fit as younger adults and are more at risk of developing physical disabilities. Primary care physicians are in a unique position to initiate preventive and rehabilitation programs for the elderly (Moore, 1978), but the effectiveness of these programs will depend on their timeliness and appropriateness. It is very important, therefore, that primary care physicians and allied health professionals understand the pathophysiology of disability in the elderly and the rationale for its prevention and treatment.

The objectives of this review are (1) to analyze the demographic factors that have led to an increasing percentage of elderly persons (and specifically women) in most of the industrialized nations, (2) present some data on the epidemiology of disability in the elderly, (3) discuss the pathophysiological basis for the prevention and treatment of disability, (4) report on the results of a few studies of the impact of physical fitness programs in elderly women, and (5) outline specific recommendations for exercise programs. Our review is limited to physical disability, although we recognize that, regardless of cause, there are important psychological and social changes that accompany a predominantly physical disability. Furthermore, we have not included in this review any studies of the impact of rehabilitation programs for specific disabilities such as stroke, which occur with great frequency in the geriatric population.

DEMOGRAPHIC CONSIDERATIONS

The population pyramid provides a useful graphic representation of the distribution of individuals in a community according to their sex and age. Different shapes of the pyramid have important implications for the organization of health care services because communities with a high proportion of elderly persons require different health facilities than communities with a predominantly young population. Figure 17.1 illustrates the striking differences in population characteristics between a developing nation like Mexico (with a high birth rate and a relatively high age-adjusted mortality) and a developed nation like Sweden (with a small birth rate and a relatively small age-adjusted death rate). The United States pyramid for 1970 is of the constricted type, showing a decreasing birth rate but still a large percentage of individuals in the young age-groups. As predicted, although not shown in Figure 17.1, the population pyramid for 1980 continues to be of the constricted type, but the median age of the U.S. population has gone up from 23 years in 1900 to 30 years in 1980. This, of course, reflects the increase in age of persons born in the late 1940s at the time that the United States experienced a so-called baby boom. Interestingly, the population pyramid for 1980 shows that 11 percent of all persons fall in the above-65 years of

FIGURE 17.1   Examples of representative population pyramids showing the increasing percentage of elderly women in industrialized nations. (Prospects for Rehabilitation of the Aged Woman. *New York Times*, 2/6/77 © 1977 by The New York Times Company. Reprinted by permission.)

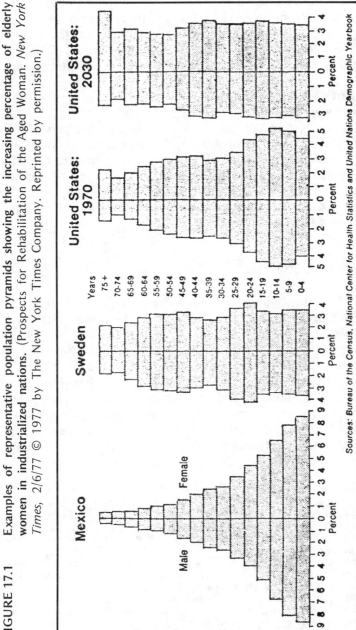

age group and that 60 percent of the elderly are women. Notwithstanding the pitfalls of projecting demographic trends of change, it is evident from Figure 17.1 that the percentage of persons above 65 years of age may increase to 20 percent by the year 2030, and that 67 percent of the elderly will be women. This projection, of course, does not take into account changes in immigration patterns.

Three factors have led to the rapidly increasing percentage of elderly women in the United States: a decrease in birth rate; a gradual decline in the age-specific death rate for persons 65 and over; and a greater survival (of approximately 8 years) for women than for men. An analysis of the causes of these profound demographic changes is beyond the scope of this review. It is clear that major medical advances and increased accessibility to health care in the last two decades have accounted in no small part for the increase in life expectancy of women.

EPIDEMIOLOGY

There is a large body of data on the magnitude of disability among elderly women. The National Center for Health Statistics (NCHS) systematically collects information about disability in the general population and specifically in elderly women through various sources: the Health Interview Survey (HIS), the Health and Nutrition Examination Survey (HANES), the National Ambulatory Medical Care Survey, and the National Nursing Home Survey. There are, of course, problems in accepting, at face value, the data provided by these sources. The scales used for determining restricted activity, although reasonably validated, may not be sufficiently sensitive or specific.[1]

---

[1] By sensitivity we mean the ability of a measurement to identify those individuals who have the characteristic or attribute being measured (true positives). For example, a test (or battery of tests) would be highly sensitive if it could identify most of the truly disabled elderly women.

By specificity we mean the ability of a measurement to detect those individuals who do not have the characteristic or attribute under measurement (true negatives). For example, a test (or battery of tests) would be highly specific if it could identify most of the elderly women who truly do not have disability.

Sensitivity and specificity are not mutually exclusive, but there are very few tests that are both highly sensitive and highly specific.

A summary of data collected in 1978 shows that 6.7 percent of persons 65 years of age and over reported having some physical limitation but not in major activities, 21 percent had limitation of major activities, and 16.6 percent were unable to carry on major activities. Thus, a total of 44.3 percent of aged persons reported some degree of physical inactivity. Of interest also is the fact that in 1978, persons 65 years of age or over had an average of 40 days of restricted activity and spent 14.5 days in bed because of disability (NCHS, 1980b). As shown in Figure 17.2, the major illnesses accounting for disability among elderly women in 1978 were arthritis and rheumatic diseases, heart disease, and hypertension. This contrasts somewhat with equivalent data for men,

FIGURE 17.2 Distribution of illnesses that cause disability in elderly men and women. (Data provided by the National Center for Health Statistics, National Center for Health Services Research: *Health United States 1978.* U.S. Department of Health, Education and Welfare Publication No. (PHS) 79-1232, Hyattsville, Md., 1979, p. 236. To some extent, a validation of the data reported by the National Center for Health Statistics has been provided by the Framingham disability study (Jette and Branch, 1981) and by a statewide analysis conducted in Massachusetts (Branch, 1977).)

Condition	Percent of persons 65 and older limited in activity	
	Female	*Male*
Arthritis and rheumatism	31.6	16.3
Heart condition	22.0	25.3
Hypertension without heart involvement	11.1	6.1
Visual impairment	8.6	7.6
Diabetes	6.4	6.2
Impairment of lower extremities and hips	5.7	4.0
Mental and nervous condition	3.8	2.0
Impairments of back and spine	3.8	2.7
Hearing impairments	2.7	2.0
Asthma	2.0	2.2

which show that heart disease was the number one disabling condition for them (NCHS, 1979a).

The data from Framingham and Massachusetts are closely similar and seem to indicate that disability may not be as prevalent among elderly men and women (noninstitutionalized) as might be inferred from data collected on a national basis (Nagi, 1976). As predicted though, the prevalence of disability (i.e., the number of disabled individuals per 100 persons of the same age-group at a given point in time) increases with age, and it is significantly greater for women than for men (Figure 17.3).

The prevalence of disability is, of course, higher among hospitalized persons. Indeed, a study conducted at Duke University (Warshaw et al., 1982) showed high percentages (30–80% depending on the age group) of persons 70 years or older who had impaired activities of daily living (decreased mobility, difficulty feeding themselves, and difficulty dressing). Tobis (1982), in commenting on these data, pointed out the need to reorganize hospital services in order to meet the needs of the growing number of elderly persons admitted to community hospitals.

Although there have been similar studies reporting on the prevalence of disability in other populations, it is extremely difficult to compare one set of data with another because of differences in the scales of measurement that have been used and in the definitions that have been adopted. As clearly pointed out in a study conducted by Henrard (1980), any measurements of disability in the elderly must consider not only physiological but also psychological and sociological dimensions, and, according to Fordyce (1982), it is equally crucial to measure what elderly persons actually do in their own milieu rather than what they can do in a different environment when submitted to a battery of standardized tests of activities of daily living. Thus, we must strive for an agreement on the specific scales of measurements that we should use to assess disability in the elderly (German, 1981). Equally important is to conduct cross-cultural studies, for only by knowing about the functional capabilities and limitations of the elderly of different countries and of different socioeconomic groups will we acquire a greater understanding of the epidemiology of disability. In this regard, we do not have any specific information about the magnitude of disability in minority elderly women.

FIGURE 17.3
Trends of increase in the prevalence of physical disability by gender and age. (From Jette & Branch, 1981. The Framingham Disability Study: II. Physical disability among the aged. *American Journal of Public Health, 71,* 1214–1216. Reproduced with permission.)

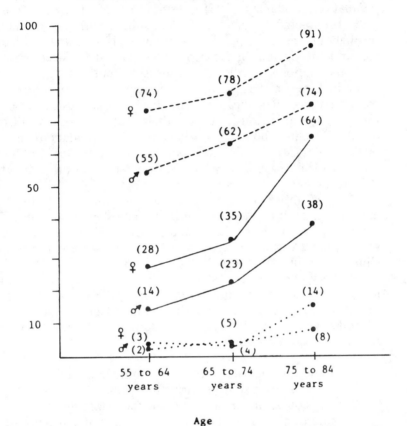

Age

----- = Difficulty in one or more physical activities

———— = Unable to perform one or more Rosow-Breslau functional health items

····· = Uses assistance in one or more activities of daily living

PHYSIOLOGICAL CONSIDERATIONS

It is well known that the process of aging is characterized by a gradual decline of the functional capacity of all organs and systems of the body. In an informative article aimed at the general population, Coughlan (1955), using data of studies by Carlson (1951), depicted the slopes of change in specific body functions throughout the life span of an individual. The data utilized to measure the decline in functional capacity of the aged are based on cross-sectional studies (i.e., measurements made at a given point in time on persons of several age-groups). It is likely that cohort studies (i.e., measurements made on groups of persons of the same age at various points in their life) would show different rates of decline, but cohort data are less abundant than cross-sectional data. In the absence of disease, it is clear that intellectual function declines later and at a slower rate than other functions (Figure 17.4).

A very noticeable early decline, and one that accounts for most physical disabilities, is that in musculoskeletal activity. Thus, from a preventive medicine and rehabilitation standpoint, we should direct our major efforts to halting and overcoming the decline in muscular function.

Primary care physicians and nurses should not recommend unnecessary bed rest and immobilization in the elderly because of the deleterious consequences that immobilization can bring to all body systems (Vallbona, 1982). Pertinent to this review is the following set of definitions:

1. Functional capacity: the maximum metabolic rate achieved by a subject during exertion.
2. Physiologic maximal potential: the maximum metabolic rate that the same individual is capable of achieving after a systematic program of physical training.
3. Functional reserve: the difference between the functional capacity and physiologic maximal potential.

Kottke (1966) discussed these concepts in a classic article dealing with the impact of immobilization and bed rest on healthy and disabled persons regardless of age. As a result of the process of aging, the functional capacity, physiologic maximal potential, and functional reserve of persons over 65 are usually lower than in

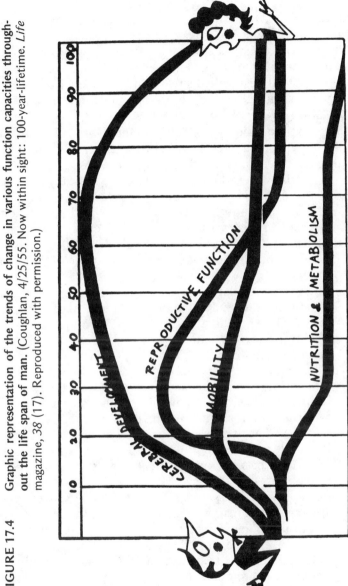

FIGURE 17.4 Graphic representation of the trends of change in various function capacities throughout the life span of man. (Coughlan, 4/25/55. Now within sight: 100-year-lifetime. *Life* magazine, *38* (17). Reproduced with permission.)

younger individuals. Elderly persons who are sedentary have a lower functional capacity than those who are active. However, a judicious program of routine continuous physical training in sedentary persons should lead to a gradual increase in their functional capacity up to a point where it may almost equal the physiologic maximal potential. On the other hand, continuing lack of exercise or prolonged bed rest will decrease the functional capacity even further and eventually the physiologic maximal potential will decrease also (Figure 17.5).

These pathophysiological concepts apply to all bodily functions, although our ability to quantitate them is greater for the muscular, cardiac, and respiratory systems. A panel of experts (de Vries, Drinkwater, Fox, Nicholas, and Smith), who participated in the 1981 National Conference on Fitness and Aging, presented abundant information about the pathophysiology of aging. A recent article written for primary care physicians summarizes the panel's reports (Fuller, 1982). The following is an excerpt of the major physiological changes identified by the panel:

1. The cardiovascular system experiences a decrease in maximum heart rate and in maximum cardiac output, and a well documented increase in arterial blood pressure.
2. The respiratory system shows a decline in vital capacity and maximum breathing capacity.
3. The musculoskeletal system exhibits a decrease in the number of muscle fibers and nerve cells, with a resultant loss of muscle strength, endurance, and coordination. The synovial fluid loses its normal viscosity, and the cartilaginous tissue becomes less elastic. These changes may render the joints more susceptible to osteoarthritis and osteoporosis. Ankylosis (locking of the joints) may become a major contributor to disability.
4. The reproductive system shows profound changes, which are most striking in women after the menopause. Probably as a result of a loss in estrogen production, postmenopausal women experience a 2% to 3% bone loss per year (4–6 times greater than that experienced by men of similar age). Thus, as the bones become very fragile, so does the risk of suffering severe fractures, which may occur spontaneously or as a result of minimal trauma. In addition, the postmenopausal decline in estrogen production accounts for an

FIGURE 17.5 **The effects of physical training and inactivity on the functional capacity of an individual.** The diagram on the left shows the levels of functional capacity, potential reserve, and maximum physiologic potential of an average person. Prolonged rest and immobilization will cause a marked decrease in functional capacity, as shown in the diagram on the bottom part of the right side. On the contrary, a program of physical exercise will increase the functional capacity and maximum physiologic potential, as shown in the top diagram of the right side of the figure. (Modified from Vallbona, 1982. Bodily responses to immobilization. In Kottke, Stillwell, & Lehmann, eds. *Krusen's Handbook of Physical Medicine and Rehabilitation* (3rd ed. pp. 963–976). Philadelphia: W. B. Saunders.)

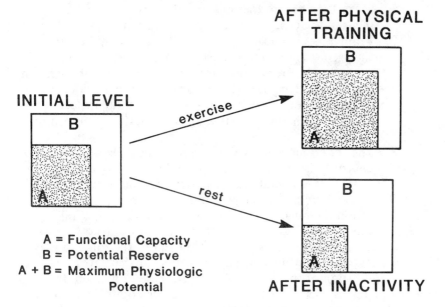

AFTER PHYSICAL TRAINING

INITIAL LEVEL

exercise

rest

A = Functional Capacity
B = Potential Reserve
A + B = Maximum Physiologic Potential

AFTER INACTIVITY

increased risk of having a myocardial infarction. Contributing to this risk and that of a stroke is the greater prevalence of hypertension among elderly women than among elderly men.

5. Oftentimes, injudicious use of medication in the elderly may contribute to a decline in functional capacity. For ex-

ample, propranolol (a beta blocker drug commonly used for the treatment of hypertension) may cause the cardiac muscle to contract less forcefully than necessary and contribute to a feeling of fatigue. Tranquilizers and other psychotropic drugs may cause excessive fatigue and somnolence.

The beneficial physiological effects of exercise in the elderly are as follows:

1. Aerobic exercise (i.e., exercise that causes oxygen demand in the muscles that does not exceed the supply) increases the amount of work performed at a given heart rate. Interestingly, after a period of training, the heart rate at rest is lower than before training, and there is an overall improvement in the efficiency of oxygen transport.
2. From a biochemical standpoint, it is likely that exercise in the aged, as in younger persons, causes a decrease in the serum level of total cholesterol and an increase in high density lipoproteins (HDL). The latter is a beneficial change since numerous studies have pointed out the protective effect of high levels of HDL against the risk of myocardial infarction.
3. The functional capacity of the musculoskeletal system also improves as a result of aerobic and anaerobic exercises. In spite of the general muscular atrophy that occurs in the elderly, there is still the possibility of increasing, through exercise, the muscle strength, range of motion, flexibility, and coordination. By submitting the bony structures to the pull of muscular contraction and to the force of gravity, important metabolic changes occur that favor remineralization of the bone tissue. In the case of women, the benefits derived from exercise may be complemented by the administration of estrogens.
4. From a general standpoint, exercise seems to promote a sense of well-being by improving the metabolic activity of the brain. An increased production of endorphins in the central nervous system after exercise may account for the greater tolerance of pain exhibited by physically active than by sedentary persons. A general elevation in mood may also result from profound biochemical changes brought about by physical activity, not unlike those

changes caused by tranquilizers or other psychotropic drugs.

IMPACT OF SPECIFIC PHYSICAL FITNESS PROGRAMS

Dacso, in the early 1950s (Dacso, 1953), had already proposed geriatric rehabilitation programs with the following goals: (1) restoration of the elderly who have an impairment in physical fitness; (2) restoration of the chronically ill without manifest signs of disability (e.g., patients with chronic cardiac or pulmonary disease); and (3) restoration of obviously handicapped persons, such as those with hemiplegia, arthritis, and so on. It would be in order to define three terms mentioned in these goals (Linn, Linn, & Wallen, 1982):

1. *Impairment* is any disturbance in any anatomical, physiological, or psychological structure or function of the body. Disturbances in the social domain may also cause an individual to have social impairments.
2. *Disability* is any decrease in functional capacity that results from the exteriorization of physiological, psychological, and social impairments. Impairments in the physiological domain may cause psychological and/or social impairments. Similarly, impairments in the psychosocial domain may lead to physiological impairments. Depending on the relative magnitude of such impairments, disability may be classified as predominantly physical, psychological, or social.
3. *Handicap* is the disadvantage that results from any disability. Thus, handicap is a comparative term that relates the disabled person to the "average normal" individual. Shortcomings of the social environment may render a disabled individual more handicapped than an equally disabled person who is capable of overcoming environmental disadvantages.

Theoretically, the prospects for physical fitness training programs in elderly women are good. Unfortunately, we do not have an abundance of published studies that document scientifically the

benefits of such programs. Cross, in an excellent review of the literature related to physical fitness training as a rehabilitation tool,
has analyzed critically the adequacy of the experimental design
and the validity of the outcomes of geriatric physical fitness training programs as reported by several authors (Cross, 1980). Studies
conducted in elderly women are those of Adams and de Vries,
(1973), Suominen, Heikkinen, and Parkatti (1977), and Gutman,
Herbert, and Brown (1977). The first two showed a beneficial
impact, while the last one reported no specific benefits.

Adams and de Vries (1973) compared an experimental group
of 17 women, who had undergone three months of vigorous physical conditioning, with a control group of 6 women. The physical
work capacity and resting heart rate of the experimental group
showed significant improvement over that of the control group.

Suominen et al. (1977) studied the impact of a varied exercise training program on men and women. There was no control
group, but 26 participants derived significant benefits from the
physical fitness regimen.

On the other hand, Gutman et al. (1977) did not find any
significant differences between a group of 32 men and women
who underwent a physical exercise program and a control group
of 35 men and women.

Unfortunately, as Cross points out, the experimental design
of the above three studies has several faults. Indeed, the number
of participants was small, and it is doubtful that those who were
placed in the experimental and in the control groups were representative of the general population of elderly women. Other
serious design flaws were insufficient information on the morbidity of the studied subjects, inadequate randomization, and questionable comparability between experimental and control groups.

In spite of similar experimental design limitations, it is pertinent to report on the study of Schuman et al. (1981) who evaluated the impact of a rehabilitation program on 229 elderly patients who had been referred to a long-term care facility over a
period of 18 months. The authors compared the outcomes of the
patients who underwent rehabilitation with those of elderly patients treated in other facilities or at home who did not participate in a structured rehabilitation program. Nondemented patients had a significantly better performance in tests of activity
of daily living three months and one year after admission to rehabilitation than those who were not admitted to the program.
Such an improvement, however, did not occur in severely demented

patients, who in some instances suffered more deterioration after rehabilitation than those equally demented patients who were not exposed to rehabilitation.

Sidney and Shephard (1977) studied the effect of 12 months of endurance training on 13 men and 21 women and reported an increase in aerobic power, favorable changes in body composition, and changes in some areas of lifestyle such as a diminished use of the car.

Lesser (1978), in a randomized experiment, assessed the effects of rhythmic exercise on the range of motion of elderly adults (mostly women) attending two nutritional centers of Maryland. She found a statistically significant improvement in the experimental group in relation to the control one.

That movement therapy may have beneficial effects beyond those of improving physiological functions was demonstrated by the study of Goldberg and Fitzpatrick (1980). They showed that a group of 30 elderly residents of a nursing home (mostly women) who participated in a supervised, albeit somewhat unspecific, movement therapy program had a statistically significant improvement in morale and attitudes toward aging when compared with a randomized control group that did not participate in the movement therapy program.

From this limited review of the impact of specific physical fitness or rehabilitation programs in elderly women, it is clear that modern geriatric medicine must adopt the rehabilitation model that has been so successful for patients with various severe physical disabilities (e.g., poliomyelitis, spinal cord injury, myocardial infarction). The model is based on the coordinated contributions of multidisciplinary teams that use various modalities of movement as therapeutic tools and that tend to address the physiological, psychological, and social needs of the disabled. Hunt (1980: p. 63) has proposed the following general guidelines for the rehabilitation of the aged:

1. Set realistic goals with the patient.
2. Allow for temporary relocation confusion.
3. Restore and maintain water and electrolyte balance.
4. Arrange priorities for drugs and schedules, to suit needed activity.
5. Search for treatable cause of instability and falls; provide stable walking aids.
6. Aim for early mobilization, always.

7. Take immediate measures to offset incontinence.
8. Use special care in assessing pain.
9. Prevent overheating.
10. Schedule active concentrated therapy for morning.
11. Keep assistive devices simple.
12. Promote community supportive services.

An additional guideline should be the establishment of ample opportunities for socialization among the elderly and between the elderly and younger adults.

More specific guidelines, of particular relevance to nurses, have been prescribed by Peters (1982).

RECOMMENDATIONS FOR PHYSICAL ACTIVITY IN THE ELDERLY

A panel of consultants from the National Council on Fitness and Aging has developed specific recommendations for exercise in the elderly (Fuller, 1982). The following is a summary:

1. Exercise should not be strenuous in order not to abuse the apparently limited physical abilities of the elderly.
2. Muscle stretching should be done routinely (warm-up) and after (cool-down) active exercises.
3. Physical fitness programs for the elderly should be supervised by physical therapists or physical educators.
4. Older athletes should be aware of their decreased faculties and exercise within the limitations of their functional potential.
5. Elderly women should participate in physical exercises as much as men.

The same panel arrived at a classification of physical activities for the elderly as follows:

1. Those that cause *too little* energy expenditure and occur too intermittently to promote endurance. Examples are light housework, walking at a rate of 1 to 2 miles per hour on level ground, playing golf using a powered cart, or bowling.

2. Those that build *moderate* endurance if carried out continuously for 15 to 30 minutes by someone of relatively
   low capacity. Activities in this group include cleaning
   windows, mopping floors, walking at a rate of 3 miles per
   hour on level ground, cycling at a rate of 6 miles per hour,
   and playing golf pulling a cart.
3. Those that promote *good* endurance if carried out for 15
   to 30 minutes. They are walking at a rate of 3½ to 4 miles
   an hour, cycling at a rate of 8 to 10 miles an hour, playing
   golf carrying clubs, skating (ice or roller), aerobic dancing,
   and swimming at a rate of less than 20 yards per minute.
5. Those that are *excellent* conditioning exercises when carried out continuously for 15 to 30 minutes. Included in
   this group are walking at a rate of 5 miles per hour, cycling at a rate of over 11 miles per hour, jogging at a rate of
   over 5½ miles an hour, and swimming at a rate of more
   than 20 yards per minute.

The above types of exercise are by no means all-inclusive.
Movement, regardless of its forms, has beneficial effects when carried out judiciously (Goldberg & Fitzpatrick, 1980). Dance, a traditional form of movement that we tend to associate with recrea-
tion, also has important therapeutic value (Hecox, Levine, &
Scott, 1976). There are also other varieties of exercise (e.g., yoga
and T'ai Chi) which until recently were not well known to physicians in the Western world and which may have a definite place in
geriatric medicine.

Physicians and allied health professionals must become thoroughly familiar with the physiological and psychological consequences of all modalities of movement, and must explore the role
that each modality may play as a part of the preventive or therapeutic armamentarium available to physicians. Each modality may
have clearly defined indications and contraindications. By knowing them, we should be in a better position to tailor preventive
or therapeutic exercise prescriptions to the needs of specific individuals, regardless of age and sex.

18
The Aged Woman and the Future of Health Care Delivery[1]

FAYE G. ABDELLAH

Who is the aged woman?

> She's anyone who is willing to admit to it in this society which battles
> wrinkles and thinks of aging females as pitiful or comic. She is anyone
> who has experienced the combined impact of age and sex discrimination
> in the job market and thinks it is about time something is done about it.
> She's one of millions of middle-aged and elderly women, the fastest
> growing population segment in this country. (DHHS, 1981)

The burdens of illness in the United States today can be traced
to lifestyle. Fifty percent of mortality from the ten leading causes
of death in the United States can be traced to lifestyle and are preventable.

Disease and disability are not inevitable events to be experienced equally by all. Each of us at birth—because of heredity,
socioeconomic background of our parents, or prenatal exposure—
may have some chance of developing a health problem.

Most serious illnesses such as heart disease and cancer are related to several factors. Some risk factors such as cigarette smoking, poor dietary habits, and severe emotional stress increase the
probabilities for several illnesses. It is the controllability of many

---

[1]Information in this paper derived from multiple sources. See Hamburg, Elliott, and
Parron, 1982; National Institute of Mental Health, 1977; U.S. Dept. of Health and
Human Services, 1980, 1981; U.S. Dept. of Health, Education and Welfare, 1978a,
1979b, 1980.

risk factors and the significance of controlling only a few that is integral to disease prevention and health promotion. A reality we face today is that the problems of old age in America are largely the problems of women. By the year 2000 there will be ten women for every five men over the age of 75. Women in the 65 and older age-group are the fastest growing segment of the U.S. population—13.9 million older women and 9.5 million older men (1977), expected to increase to 33.4 million women and 22.4 million men by the year 2035. Thus, by the year 2050 a 65-year-old woman can expect to live to the age of 85.7 or 5.7 years longer than her male counterpart.

There are also differences between the life expectancy rate for black women. In 1974, it was 71.2 years for black women and 76.6 years for white women (a difference of 5.4 years). The profile of leading causes of death is quite similar for black and white women with the exception that deaths from homicide appear in the ten leading causes of death for black women.

The key objective in addressing the future of health care delivery particularly for older women is to increase the number who can function independently and stay out of institutions. Older women hope for a state of well-being that will allow them to perform at their highest functional capacity on physical, psychological, and social levels. Their greatest fear is of being helpless, useless, sick, or unable to care for themselves.

Most elderly Americans can and do remain in their own homes —only 5 percent live in institutions. Our research in the Public Health Service showed that the average older woman at home had as many as three chronic conditions, but the dysfunctions of incontinence and senility were the driving forces that institutionalized them.

We also know that the majority of elderly women are relatively healthy and independent. Activity limitations include mental disabilities, heart conditions, arthritis and rheumatism, hearing loss, and visual impairments.

The underlying fact is that a greater proportion of the elderly could maintain a relatively independent lifestyle and vastly improve the quality of their lives. Growing old does not mean that severe physical and mental decline in aged women is inevitable. It is estimated that about half of the nation's one million elderly living in long-term care institutions are there because they were diagnosed as senile, and the diagnosis is not always justified. It is common to learn of a mistaken diagnosis because physicians and families attribute mental decline and behavioral change associated with physical conditions to senility and fail to initiate appropriate and timely treatment.

Many causes of apparent senility can be treated to reverse the condition. Such causes include drug interaction, depression, metabolic disorders (thyroid, kidney, liver, and pituitary malfunctions), chronic subdural hematoma, certain tumors, alcohol toxicities, chemical intoxications (arsenic, mercury, aluminum), nutritional deficiencies, sensory deprivation due to failing sight and hearing, incontinence, and anemia.

Obviously the reversible mental impairments are numerous. Even with irreversible organic brain syndrome, measures are available to lessen patient discomfort and to slow or arrest deterioration.

One cannot emphasize enough that attention needs to be given to the potentially adverse effects of the many and varied drugs prescribed for the elderly. The average older woman who is institutionalized has as many as five different tranquilizers prescribed for her. The physiological absorption and excretion patterns of drugs taken by women 65 and over is much slower and the effects often lead to unanticipated drug interactions.

The mental confusion of aged women, often attributed to senility, can be minimized if they have access to a continuing, well-informed source of health care and patient/client education. Among the most frequent chronic conditions and impairments of older women in the community are arthritis (44% of those over 65), reduced vision (22%), hearing impairments (29%), heart conditions (20%), and hypertension (35%).

The aged woman on the average is limited to restricted activity 5.5 weeks a year. As much as one-third of this is due to acute illness or injuries. Such acute episodes as burns, falls, influenza, or pneumonia can be prevented.

We have learned of the importance of finding the sick and disabled in the population early to help them. Such community outreach programs as are being conducted in Texas have proved to be highly successful in reducing the number of hospitalizations of older people.

Early screening and detection programs using patient/client assessment techniques can help to identify and treat such conditions as glaucoma, hypertension, some types of anemia, depression, hearing disorders, some cancers, and overmedication.

A comprehensive and integrated system of geriatric services provided in a single location can be most effective in carrying out health surveillance and health maintenance.

Fear of the cost of severe illness may cause aged women to conserve their limited resources. Cheap foods and housing and fear itself prevent them from leading full and active lives.

Exercise and fitness for older women need to be stressed. Movement is critical to functional living. The quality of intellectual and physical performances is enhanced by becoming and remaining physically and mentally active.

RESEARCH

More research is needed on aged women including research that addresses important methodological issues.

Methodological Issues

- More data are needed about women as individuals. Major data sources such as the Bureau of the Census deal with women as wives, mothers, or heads of households.
- Longitudinal data are needed about women as they move in and out of the labor force.
- More information is needed about families—family network and family structures.
- Data are needed on minority women, such as women of specific ethnic groups and social classes, rural women, and childless women.
- Longitudinal studies of women's lives linked to relevant social, economic, and political events are also needed.

Health and Illness

The following topics are ripe for further investigation.

- Osteoporosis—the decrease of bone mass or "thinning" usually diagnosed following common fractures of the hip, wrist, vertebrae. Causes suggested are lower levels of estrogen, loss of calcium, and smoking and caffeine.
- Treatable loss of vision, hearing, mobility, and levels of nutrition.
- Prevention, early detection, and treatment of all kinds of cancer.

- Cryptogenic drop attacks that contribute to the rate of bone fractures.
- Stress incontinence and the effectiveness of biofeedback techniques for both the ambulatory and institutionalized aged woman.

Senile Dementias

- There is a need for the study of the effects on physical and mental health of interacting biological, psychological, and social factors.
- Epidemiological data about prevalence in aged women of pseudodementia, treatable brain syndrome, alcoholism, medication use and abuse must be collected.
- Alzheimer's disease needs further investigation.
- It would be helpful to confirm findings in senile dementia of a reduction of choline acetyl transferase (CAT)—the enzyme essential to synthesize acetyl choline, which transmits information within the brain.
- A study should be mounted to confirm that secondary hyperparathyroidism caused by lack of calcium and magnesium in the environment provokes an accumulation of metal ions in brain tissue, such as aluminum.
- A core question in research of the aged woman is the degree to which a change in function or biochemistry of an aging tissue is due to shifts in the mixture of cell types or to alteration in individual cells. Such advances as monoclonal antibodies and other identification techniques may help determine the specific cellular components in aging tissues.

Prevention

- Effective systems for teaching the elderly to cope with the aging process must be developed. Exploration needs to be done of ways of finding and applying effective strategies for disseminating information about prevention through the media, educational institutions, health care providers, senior citizens groups, and the like.

Epilogue: Prospects for Treatment and Research

In the process of examining the physical and mental health of aged women from diverse perspectives, several promising suggestions and proposals for improved treatment and prevention have been advanced in individual chapters. Where a specific treatment is at present lacking, there are still some clues for research. This final chapter, therefore, will summarize the prospects for treatment and prevention and identify major research questions that will need to be addressed before we can effectively improve the lot of aged women.

PROSPECTS FOR TREATMENT AND PREVENTION

Guidelines for health maintenance and the treatment of health problems characteristic of elderly women can be roughly divided into three categories: medical or surgical therapy, the provision and use of services, and psychosocial interventions.

Medical and Surgical Therapy

Long overdue attention is being focused today on the use and abuse of drugs among the elderly, taking note of the fact that the prescription of drugs for elderly women exceeds that for elderly men. More knowledge about the pharmacokinetics, pharmacodynamics, and side effects of drugs in the elderly is making possible more rational use of these substances. "Polypharmacy" (the use of multiple drugs), usually an inadvertent by-product of our fragmented health care system, has come to be recognized as a major threat to the health of older women, who often suffer from multiple health problems. Most of what we are currently learning about drugs in the elderly points toward the prescription and use of a smaller number of drugs and smaller doses of those that are used (see Chapter 15 by Hoppel).

One of the most disabling disorders in the postmenopausal woman is shown by Lindsay in Chapter 5 to be osteoporosis. A hopeful development in this field is the increasingly scientific basis for the use of replacement estrogen and supplemental calcium, as described in that chapter. An even more enthusiastic endorsement of the use of replacement hormone therapy is given in Chapter 6 by Greenblatt and colleagues, although it may be well at this point to introduce a note of caution, since there is far from universal agreement today that benefits of such use of estrogens outweigh the risks.

Welch, in Chapter 14, gives a clear presentation of the most common health problems of older women that can be effectively improved with surgery. Currently, new approaches to the evaluation of surgical outcome hold the promise that such techniques as cost/benefit analysis and decision-trees can permit us to apply information from extensive past experience to systematic and logical decision making about the probability of a successful outcome in a patient characterized by specific risk factors (Bunker, Barnes, & Mosteller, 1977).

Provision and Use of Services

Somers (Chapter 2) reminds us of the very great increase in federal funding of health services for older persons that has taken place since the introduction of Medicare and Medicaid in 1965. In the light of increasing population and shrinking resources, it seems unlikely that further public payment for health and social services will be possible in the immediate future, and it will be a task just to maintain the progress already made. Nevertheless, it is well to bear in mind that older women do, in fact, have much better access to care than in the past (Rogers, Blendon, & Moloney, 1982). Better provision of rehabilitation services, in particular, is beginning to be recognized as a high priority for the numerous older women (and men) who suffer strokes, hip fractures, and other physically disabling events (see Chapter 17 by Vallbona).

Along with improved public financing during the past two decades, there has been a striking growth of the nursing home system in the United States. Although only about 5 percent of older persons live in nursing homes, more than a quarter of those who reach the age of 65 in this country will die in a nursing home (Katz, Zdeb, & Therriault, 1979). Partly because of our financing system, we have opted for nursing home placement as the solution to numerous kinds of care problems. We are now beginning to recognize the impact of the institutional environment and to give active attention to alternatives to nursing home placement (see Chapter 16 by Kahana and Kahana). Older women are understandably preoccupied with the balance between desired independence and the need for a reliable support system. Current trends suggest that in the future they will have more options from which to choose living arrangements adapted to their individual needs.

Psychosocial Intervention

In several chapters, notably Chapter 18 by Abdellah and Chapter 1 by Riley, it has been pointed out that we are now in a position to make documented recommendations about improved health habits, about learning how to cope with age-related stresses, and about how to achieve better nutrition (see Chapter 13 by Mitchell). Beyond these rather pragmatic forms of health maintenance there lies the possibility that a better understanding of nutrition may contribute to the prevention of cancer (Doll, 1977).

In terms of mental health, the current move toward clearer definitions of dementia and depression has already made possible improvement in the diagnosis and treatment of these conditions (see Chapter 7 by Holzer). In addition, Gutman, in Chapter 8, points to encouraging evidence that psychological and social growth and development are possible for older women, and, in specific social circumstances, are almost routine. Major changes in the demography and social roles of women in general and older women in particular have been commented on by several contributors. Although the ultimate impact of these changes is mainly a matter for future research, there are suggestions that better support systems *for* women, as opposed to existing support systems which depend largely upon women themselves, may be in the process of developing. An additional hopeful note is struck by Riley's suggestion that technological development may really work to the advantage of older women.

MAJOR RESEARCH QUESTIONS

In almost every chapter, suggestions for future research have been mentioned or elaborated upon. We have selected three major questions to summarize the need for more intensive investigation in this field.

Why Do Women Live Longer Than Men?

The strikingly greater life expectancy that women now enjoy, as compared to men, is a very recent historical development. In the past, the risks and trauma associated with repetitive childbearing prior to the advent of modern obstetrics meant that women rarely outlived their spouses. Now that the morbidity and mortality associated with childbirth have been greatly reduced, we are faced with the intriguing new problem of women's superior survival. Can this be attributed to some intrinsic or socially conditioned strength of the female sex? There may be a clue to what this quality is that could be discovered in the study of aged black women. As Somers points out in Chapter 2, black women of 65 and over have extraordinarily high life expectancies. What makes these "survivors" so rugged? One obvious channel of investigation is along the line of hormonal differences, while a recent explosion of information about the immune system may suggest another basis for long life among women. Can the sex differences, on the other hand, be explained by some inherent weakness or unfavorable pattern of stress related to work and social interaction among men? A good possibility for resolving this question is offered by the impending cohort of more divorced, single, working women who are increasingly assuming a "masculine" lifestyle. The hypothesis that stress, in one of its numerous forms, shortens men's lives could be tested in a prospective study of the new generation of women who will be aging in the next decade or two, compared with their male contemporaries.

Why Are All Elderly Surviving Longer?

The remarkable and unpredicted trend toward dramatic improvement in life expectancy among the very old has been recognized so recently that research approaches to its study have scarcely been formulated. One hypothesis, suggested by Somers in Chapter 2, is that improved access to health services since the introduction of federal funding of care for the aged is an underlying factor. This change alone, however, does not explain why the reduction in mortality has been principally in the cardiovascular diseases. Extremely aged women continue to experience lower mortality than do men of the same age, but the sex differences are less than in the past (Rosenwaike, Yaffe, & Sagi, 1980). A full understanding of the greatly improved health and longevity being experienced today by older American women will have to be consistent with a general explanation of this phenomenon as it applies to both sexes.

What Will Be the Impact of the Changing Character of the Family and the Changing Role of Women?

Finally, we return to some of the research questions raised in the initial chapter, by Riley. What lies ahead for the present cohort of aging women, so different from their predecessors? The rising curve of labor force participation by women, changing sex roles, smaller families, increased divorce rate, plus increased longevity seem to be leading to a society with an extraordinarily high proportion of widowed or divorced elderly women, bereft of kin, in reasonably good health, but potentially socially isolated. Research is surely needed to define the appropriate financial, social, housing, and psychological support systems they will need.

Ironically, the position of the aged woman today might be classified as an example of what Gruenberg has called "the failures of success," success being the improved longevity that we have already seen, and the "failures" being the many problems detailed in this book (Gruenberg, 1977). Can we find successful solutions to these new problems as well?

M. R. Haug
A. B. Ford
M. Sheafor

References and Bibliography

Abrahams, R. B. (1972). Mutual help for the wodowed. *Social Work, 17*, 54–61.

Adams, B. N. (1968). *Kinship in an urban setting*. Chicago: Markham.

Adams, G. M., & de Vries, H. A. (1973). Physiological effects of an exercise training regimen upon women aged 52 to 79. *Journal of Gerontology, 28*, 50–55.

Agee, J. M. (1980). Grief and the process of aging. In J. A. Werner-Belend (Ed.), *Grief responses to long-term illness and disability* (pp. 133–168). Reston, VA: Reston.

Albanese, A. A. (1978). Calcium nutrition in the elderly: Maintaining bone health to minimize fracture risk. *Postgraduate Medicine, 63*, 167–172.

Albright, F., Blomberg, E., & Smith, P. H. (1940). Postmenopausal osteoporosis. *Transactions of the Association of American Physicians, 55*, 298–305.

Allan C., & Brotman, B. (1981). *Chartbook on aging in America*. Washington, DC: White House Conference on Aging.

Aloia, J. F., Cohn, S. H., Ostuni, J. A., Cane, R., & Ellis, K. (1978). Prevention of involutional bone loss by exercise. *Annals of Internal Medicine, 89*, 356–358.

Alyward, M. (1973). Plasma tryptophan levels and mental depression in postmenopausal subjects. Effects of oral piperazine-oestrone sulphate. *Medical Science, 1*, 30.

American Psychiatric Association. (1980). *Diagnostic and statistical manual of mental disorders* (3rd ed.). Washington, DC: Author.

Anderson, N. N. (1974). Approaches to improving the quality of long-term care for older persons. *Gerontologist, 14*, 519–524.

Andres, R., & Tobin, J. D. (1975). Aging and the disposition of glucose. In V. J. Cristofalo, J. Roberts, & R. C. Adelman (Eds.), *Exploration in Aging: Advances and Experiment in Medicine and Biology, 61*, 239–249.

Archbold, P. G. (1980). *Impact of parent-caring on women*. Unpublished doctoral dissertation, University of California, San Francisco.

Archbold, P. G. (1982). All-consuming activity: The family as caregiver. *Generations, Winter*, 12–13.

Arling, G. (1976). Resistance to isolation among elderly widows. *International Journal of Aging and Human Development, 7*, 67–86.

Avioli, L. V. (1981). Postmenopausal osteoporosis: Prevention versus cure. *Federation Proceedings, 40*(9), 2418–2422.

Avioli, L. V., McDonald, J. E., & Lee, S. W. (1965). The influence of age on the intestinal absorption of 47-Ca in women and its relationship to 47-Ca absorption in postmenopausal osteoporosis. *The Journal of Clinical Investigations, 44,* 1960–1967.

Azizi, F., Vagenakis, A. G., Portnay, G. I., Rapoport, B., Ingber, S., Braverman, L. E. (1975). Pituitary-thyroid responsiveness to intramuscular thyrotropin-releasing hormone based on analyses of serum thyrotoxine, tri-iodothyronine, and thyrotropin concentrations. *New England Journal of Medicine, 299,* 273–277.

Babchuk, N. (1978). Aging and primary relations. *Aging and Human Development, 9,* 137–151.

Bahr, H. M. (1976). The kinship role. In F. I. Nye (Ed.), *Role structure and analysis of the family* (pp. 61–79). Vol. 24, Sage Library of Social Research. Beverly Hills: Sage.

Bahr, H. M., & Nye, F. I. (1974). The kinship role in a contemporary community: Perceptions of obligations and sanctions. *Journal of Comparative Family Studies, 5*(Spring), 17–25.

Barlow, J. J., Emerson, K., & Saxena, B. N. (1969). Estradiol production after ovariectomy for carcinoma of the breast. *New England Journal of Medicine, 270,* 633–637.

Barton, E. M., Baltes, M. M., & Orzech, M. J. (1980). Etiology of dependence in older nursing home residents during morning care: The role of staff behavior. *Journal of Personality and Social Psychology, 38,* 423–431.

Beck, A. J. (1973). *The diagnosis and management of depression.* Philadelphia: University of Pennsylvania Press.

Beck, P. (1982). Two successful interventions in nursing homes: The therapeutic effects of cognitive activity. *Gerontologist, 22,* 378–383.

Beeson, D. (1975). Women in studies of aging: A critique and suggestion. *Social Problems, 23,* 52–59.

Behavior Today. (1979, April). 10.

Belloc, N. B. (1973). Relationship of health practices and mortality. *Preventive Medicine, 2,* 67–81.

Belloc, N. B., & Breslow, L. (1972). Relationship of physical health status and health practices. *Preventive Medicine, 1,* 409–421.

Bengtson, V., & Black, O. (1973). Intergenerational relations: Continuities in socialization. In P. Baltes & W. Schaie (Eds.), *Life span developmental psychology: Personality and Socialization* (pp. 207–234). New York: Academic.

Bengtson, V., Kasschau, L., & Ragan, P. K. (1977). The impact of social structure on aging individuals. In J. E. Birren & K. Schaie (Eds.), *Handbook of the psychology of aging* (pp. 327–353). New York: Van Nostrand Reinhold.

Bennett, R., & Eisdorfer, C. (1975). The institutional environment and behavior change. In S. Sherwood (Ed.), *Long-term care: A handbook for researchers, planners, and providers* (pp.391–453). New York: Spectrum.

Berardo, F. M. (1967). Kinship interaction and communication among space-age immigrants. *Journal of Marriage and the Family, 29,* 541–554.

Berkman, L. F., & Syme, S. L. (1979). Social networks, host resistance, and mortality: A nine-year follow-up study of Alameda County residents. *American Journal of Epidemiology, 109,* 186–204.

Berkman, P. L. (1975). Survival, and a modicum of indulgence in the sick role. *Medical Care, 13,* 85–94.

Bistrian, B. R., Blackburn, G. L., Vitale, J., Cochran, D., & Naylor, J. (1976). Prevalence of malnutrition in general medical patients. *Journal of the American Medical Association, 235,* 1567–1570.

Black, E. R. (1980). Use of special aids, United States, 1977. *Vital and Health Statistics, Series 10,* No. 135 (DHHS Publication No. PHS 81-1563). Hyattsville, MD: National Center for Health Statistics.

Blazer, D., & Williams, C. D. (1980). Epidemiology of dysphoria and depression in an elderly population. *American Journal of Psychiatry, 137,* 439–444.

Blenkner, M. (1967). Environmental change and the aging individual. *Gerontologist, 7* (2, pt. I.), 101–105.

Blichert-Toft, M. (1978). The adrenal glands in old age. In R. B. Greenblatt (Ed.), *Aging* (Vol. 1). *Geriatric endocrinology.* New York: Raven.

Blichert-Toft, M., Blichert-Toft, B., & Jensen, H. K. (1970). Pituitary-adrenocortical stimulation in the aged as reflected in levels of plasma cortisol and compound S. *Acta Chirurgica Scandinavica, 136,* 665–670.

Block, J., von der Lippe, A., & Block, J. H. (1973). Sex-role and socialization patterns: Some personality concomitants and environmental antecedents. *Journal of Consulting and Clinical Psychology, 41,* 321–341.

Block, M. R., Davidson, J. L., & Grambs, J. D. (1981). *Women over forty: Visions and realities.* New York: Springer.

Bornstein, P. E., Clayton, P. J., Halikas, J. A., Maurice, W. L., & Robins, E. (1973). The depression of widowhood after thirteen months. *The British Journal of Psychiatry, 122,* 561–566.

Botwinick, J., & Storandt, M. (1980). Recall and recognition of old information in relation to age and sex. *Journal of Gerontology, 35,* 70–76.

Bourestom, N. C., & Pastalan, L. (1972). *Relocation reports 1 and 2.* Ann Arbor, MI: Institute of Gerontology, University of Michigan.

Bowlby, J. (1961). Process of mourning. *The International Journal of Psychoanalysis, 42,* 317–340.

Branch, L. G. (1977). Updating the needs of the Massachusetts elderly. *New England Journal of Medicine, 297,* 838–840.

Branch, L. G., & Jette, A. M. (1981). The Framingham Disability Study: I. Social disability among the aging. *American Journal of Public Health, 71,* 1202–1210.

Brickel, C. M. (1979). The therapeutic roles of cat mascot with a hospital-based geriatric population: A staff survey. *Gerontologist, 19,* 368–372.

Brock, E. W., & Webber, I. L. (1972). Suicide among the elderly: Isolating widowhood and mitigating alternatives. *Journal of Marriage and the Family, 34,* 24–31.

Brody, E. M. (1978). The aging of the family. *The Annals of the American Academy of Political and Social Science* [Special issue, E. Wolfgang & R. Lambert (Eds.), "Planning for the elderly."] *438*, 13–27.

Brody, E. M. (1982). "Women in the middle" and family help to older people. *Gerontologist, 21*, 471–480.

Brody, J. A., & Brock, D. B. (in press). Epidemiological and statistical characteristics of the United States elderly population. In C. E. Finch & E. L. Schneider (Eds.), *Handbook of the biology of aging* (2nd ed.). New York: Van Nostrand Reinhold.

Brotman, H. B. (1982). *Every ninth American: An analysis for the Chairman of the Select Committee on Aging, House of Representatives, 97th Congress, 2nd Session.* Washington, DC: U.S. Government Printing Office.

Bulbrook, R. D., & Greenwood, F. C. (1957). Persistence of urinary oestrogen excretion after oophorectomy and adrenalectomy. *British Medical Journal, I*, 662–668.

Bullamore, J. R., Gallagher, J. C., Wilkinson, R., Nordin, B. E. C., & Marshall, D. H. (1970). Effect of age on calcium absorption. *Lancet, ii*, 535–537.

Bunker, J. P., Barnes, B. A., & Mosteller, F. (Eds.). (1977). *Costs, risks, and benefits of surgery.* New York: Oxford University Press.

Burnside, I. M. (1969). Grief work in the aged patient. *Nursing Forum, 8*, 416–427.

Burnside, I. M. (1982). *The concept of hallucinations.* Unpublished manuscript.

Busse, E. W. (1978). How mind, body, and environment influence nutrition in the elderly. *Postgraduate Medicine, 63*, 118–125.

Bustad, L., & Hines, L. (1982). Placement of animals with the elderly: Benefits and strategies. *California Veterinarian, 36*(8), 36–44.

Bustad, L. K. (1980). *Animals, aging, and the aged.* Minneapolis: University of Minnesota Press.

Butler, R. N. (1963). The life review: An interpretation of reminiscence in the aged. *Psychiatry, 26*, 65–76.

Butler, R. N. (1975). Psychiatry and the elderly: An overview. *American Journal of Psychiatry, 132*, 893–900.

Butler, R. N., & Lewis, M. (1977). Aging and mental health: *Positive psychosocial approaches* (2nd ed.). St Louis: C. V. Mosby.

Caine, L. (1974). *Widow.* New York: Morrow.

Caine, L. (1978). *Lifelines.* New York: Doubleday.

Carlson, A. J. (1951). Physiologic changes in aging. *Quarterly Bulletin Northwestern University Medical School, 25*, 392–395.

Carp, F. M. (1975). Impact of improved housing on morale and life satisfaction. *Gerontologist, 15*, 511–515.

Carter, A. C. (1982). Religion and the black elderly: The historical basis of social and psychological concerns. In R. C. Manuel (Ed.), *Minority aging: Sociological and social psychological issues* (pp. 103–108). Westport, CT: Greenwood.

Chestnut, C. H., III, Ivey, J. L., Nelp, W. B., & Baylink, D. J. (1979). An assessment of anabolic steroids and calcitonin in the treatment of osteoporosis. In U.S. Barzel (Ed.), *Osteoporosis II* (pp. 135–150). New York: Grune & Stratton.

Chevan, A., & Korson, J. H. (1972). The widowed who live alone: An examination of social and demographic factors. *Social Forces, 51,* 45–53.

Chodorow, N. (1978). *The reproduction of mothering: Psychoanalysis and the sociology of gender.* Berkeley: University of California Press.

Christiansen, C., Christiansen, M. S., & Transbøl, I. (1981). Bone mass in postmenopausal women after withdrawal of oestrogen/gestagen replacement therapy. *Lancet, i,* 459–461.

Clayton, P. J. (1973). The clinical morbidity of the first year of bereavement: A review. *Comprehensive Psychiatry, 14,* 151–157.

Clayton, P. J. (1975). The effects of living alone on bereavement symptoms. *American Journal of Psychiatry, 132,* 133–137.

Cleveland, W. P., & Gianturco, D. T. (1976). Remarriage probability after widowhood: A retrospective method. *Journal of Gerontology, 31,* 99–103.

Clymer, A. (1982, June 30). Women's political habits show sharp change. *New York Times,* pp. A1, D22.

Cobb, S. (1979). Social support and health through the life course. In AAAS Selected Symposium 30, *Aging from birth to death: Interdisciplinary perspectives,* (Vol. 1, pp. 93–106). Boulder, CO: Westview.

Coe, R. M. (1965). Self-conception and institutionalization. In A. M. Rose & W. A. Peterson (Eds.), *Older people and their social world: The subculture of aging.* Philadelphia: F. A. Davis.

Coe, R. M., & Brehm, H. P. (1972). *Preventive health care for adults: A study of medical practice.* New Haven, CT: College & University Press.

Coles, R. (1975). *The old ones of New Mexico.* Garden City, NY: Anchor.

Cooke, J. N. C., James, V. H. T., Landon, J., & Wynn, V. (1964). Adrenocortical function in chronic malnutrition. *British Medical Journal, I,* 662–666.

Costello, J. P., & Tanaka, G. M. (1961). Mortality and morbidity in long-term institutional care of the aged. *Journal of the American Geriatrics Society, 9,* 959–966.

Coughlan, R. (1955, April 25). Now within sight: 100-year-lifetime. *Life* magazine, *38*(17), 156–158, 160, 162, 165–169, 170–173.

Crandall, R. C. (1980). *Gerontology: A behavioral science approach.* Reading, MA: Addison-Wesley.

Cross, D. L. (1980). The influence of physical fitness training as a rehabilitation tool. *International Journal of Rehabilitation Research, 3,* 163–175.

Dacso, M. M. (1953). Clinical problems in geriatric rehabilitation. *Geriatrics, 8,* 179–185.

de Castillejo, I. C. (1973). *Knowing woman: A feminine psychology.* New York: Harper and Row.

Deftos, L. J., Weisman, M. H., Williams, G. W., Karpf, D. B., Frumar, A. M., Davidson, B. J., Parthemore, J. G., & Judd, H. L. (1980). Influence of age and sex on plasma calcitonin in human beings. *New England Journal of Medicine, 302*: 1351–1353.

Dennerstein, L., Laby, B., Burrows, G. D., & Hyman, G. J. (1978). Headache and sex hormone therapy. *Headache, 18*, 146–153.

Denney, N. N. (1980). Task demands and problem solving strategies in middle-aged and older adults. *Journal of Gerontology, 35*, 559–664.

De Vita, V. T., Jr. (1980, September 26). Statement before the Select Committee on Aging. House of Representatives. *Research frontiers in aging and cancer. International symposium for the 1980s.* Committee Pub. No. 96-275. Washington, DC: U.S. Government Printing Office.

DeWever, M. K. (1977). Nursing home patients' perception of nurses' affective touching. *Journal of Psychology, 96*, 163–171.

Doherty, E. G. (1978). Are differential discharge criteria used for men and women psychiatric inpatients. *Journal of Health and Social Behavior, 19*, 107–116.

Doll, R. (1977). Strategy for detection of cancer hazards. *Nature, 265*, 589–596.

Donaldson, G. A., & Welch, C. E. (1968). Urgent surgery: Abdominal emergencies. In J. H. Powers (Ed.), *Surgery of the aged and debilitated patient* (pp. 372–404). Philadephia: Saunders.

Dothard v. Rawlinson, 433 U.S. 321 (M. D. Ala., 1977).

Dowd, J. J., & Bengtson, V. (1978). Aging in minority populations: An examination of the double jeopardy hypothesis. *Journal of Gerontology, 33*, 427–436.

Dunphy, J. E. (1968). Elective surgery in old age. In J. H. Powers (Ed.), *Surgery of the aged and debilitated patient* (pp. 350–371). Philadelphia: Saunders.

Dye, C. J., & Erber, J. T. (1981). Two group procedures for the treatment of nursing home patients. *Gerontologist, 21*, 539–544.

Evans, A. W. H., Woodrow, J. C., McDougall, C. D. M., Chew, A. R., & Evans, R. W. (1967). Antibodies in the families of thyrotoxic patients. *Lancet, i*, 636–641.

Falletti, M. V. (1982). Human factors research and functional environments for the aged. In I. Altman, J. Wohlwill, & M. P. Lawton (Eds.), *Human behavior and environment: Advances in theory and research* (Vol. 7). New York: Plenum.

Felton, B., & Kahana, E. (1974). Adjustment and situationally bound locus of control among institutionalized aged. *Journal of Gerontology, 29*, 295–301.

Fenyö, G. (1982). Acute abdominal disease in the elderly: Experience from two series in Stockholm. *American Journal of Surgery, 143*, 751–754.

Fingerhut, L. A. (1982). Changes in mortality among the elderly: United States, 1940–78. *Vital and Health Statistics, Series 3*, No. 22 (DHHS Publication No. PHS 82-1406). Washington, DC: U.S. Government Printing Office.

Folstein, M. F., Folstein, S. E., & McHugh, P. R. (1975). Mini-Mental State: A practical method for grading the cognitive state of patients for the clinician. *Journal of Psychiatric Research, 12,* 189–198.

Fordyce, W. E. (1982). Geriatric patients [letter]. *Archives of Physical Medicine and Rehabilitation, 63,* 290.

Friedman, E. (1979). Pet ownership and survival after coronary heart diseases. *Proceedings of Second Canadian Symposium on Pets and Society,* Toronto, Canada: Dr. Ballards Pet Food, Division of Standard Brands Foods.

Friedman, M., Green, M. F., & Sharland, D. E. (1969). Assessment of hypothalamic-pituitary-adrenal function in the geriatric age group. *Journal of Gerontology, 24,* 292–297.

Fries, J. F. (1980). Aging, natural death, and the compression of morbidity. *New England Journal of Medicine, 303,* 130–135.

Fries, J. F., & Crapo, L. M. (1981). *Vitality and aging: Implications of the rectangular curve.* San Francisco: W. H. Freeman.

Frontera v. Sindell, 522 F. 2d 1215 (6th Cir. 1975).

Fuller, E. (1982). Exercise: Getting the elderly going. *Patient Care, 16,* 67–114.

Fuxe, K. (1964). Cellular localization of monoamines in the median eminence and infundibular stem of some mammals. *Zeitschrift fur Zellforschung und Mikroskopische Anatomie, 61,* 710–724.

Gambrell, R. D., Jr. (1978). The prevention of endometrial cancer in postmenopausal women with progestins. *Maturitas, 1,* 107–112.

Garraway, W. M., Stauffer, R. N., Kurland, L. T., & O'Fallon, W. M. (1979). Limb fractures in a defined population. 1. Frequency and distribution. *Mayo Clinic Proceedings, 54,* 701–707.

Genant, H. T., Heck, L. L., Lanzl, L. H., Rossmann, K., Horst, J. V., & Paloyan, E. (1973). Primary hyperparathyroidism: A comprehensive study of clinical, biochemical, and radiographic manifestations. *Radiology, 109,* 513–524.

Geokas, M. C., & Haverback, B. J. (1969). The aging gastrointestinal tract. *American Journal of Surgery, 117,* 881–889.

George, L. K. (1980). *Role transitions in later life.* Monterey, CA: Brooks/ Cole.

Gerber, I., Rusalem, R., Hannon, N., Battin, D., & Arkin, A. (1975). Anticipatory grief and aged widows and widowers. *Journal of Gerontology, 30,* 225–229.

German, P. S. (1981). Measuring functional disability in the older population. *American Journal of Public Health, 71,* 1197–1199.

Gibbs, J. M. (1974). *Role changes associated with widowhood among middle and upper class women.* Paper presented at the meeting of the Midwest Sociological Society, Omaha, NB.

Gilligan, C. (1982). *In a different voice: Psychological theory and women's development.* Cambridge, MA: Harvard University Press.

Goffman, E. (1961). *Asylums: Essays on the social situation of mental patients and other inmates.* Garden City, NY: Doubleday.

Goldberg, W. G., & Fitzpatrick, J. J. (1980). Movement therapy with the aged. *Nursing Research, 29,* 339–346.

Goldfarb, A. I. (1969). Predicting mortality in the institutionalized aged. *Archives of General Psychiatry, 21,* 172–176.

Goldman, R. (1979). Decline in organ function with aging. In I. Rossman (Ed.), *Clinical geriatrics* (2nd ed., pp. 23–59). Philadelphia: Lippincott.

Gottesman, L. E., & Bourestom, N. C. (1974). Why nursing homes do what they do. *Gerontologist, 14,* 501–506.

Gramlich, E. P. (1968). Recognition and management of grief in elderly patients. *Geriatrics, 23,* 87–92.

Grattarola, R., Secreto, G., & Recchione, C. (1975). Correlation between urinary testosterone or estrogen excretion levels and interstitial cell-stimulating hormone concentrations in normal postmenopausal women. *American Journal of Obstetrics and Gynecology, 121:* 380–381.

Greenblatt, D. J. (1979). Reduced serum albumin concentration in the elderly: A report from the Boston Collaborative Drug Surveillance Program. *Journal of the American Geriatrics Society, 27,* 20–22.

Greenblatt, D. J., Sellers, E. M., & Shader, R. I. (1982). Drug disposition in old age. *New England Journal of Medicine, 306,* 1081–1088.

Greenblatt, R. B., Barfield, W. E., Garner, J. F., Calk, G. Y., & Harrod, J. P., Jr. (1950). Evaluation of an estrogen, androgen, estrogen-androgen combination, and a placebo in the treatment of menopause. *Journal of Clinical Endocrinology, 10,* 1547–1558.

Greenblatt, R. B., Colle, M. L., & Mahesh, V. B. (1976). Ovarian and adrenal steroid production in the postmenopausal woman. *Obstetrics and Gynecology, 47,* 383–387.

Greenblatt, R. B., Nezhat, C., Roesel, R. A., & Natrajan, P. K. (1979). Update on the male and female climacteric. *Journal of the American Geriatrics Society, 27,* 481–490.

Greenblatt, R. B., & Rose, F. D. (1962). Delay of menses: Test of progestational efficacy in induction of pseudopregnancy. *Obstetrics and Gynecology, 19,* 730–735.

Greenblatt, R. B., Stoddard, L. D., & King, P. R. (1966). Estrogen in endometrial carcinogenesis. In G. C. Lewis, Jr., W. B. Wentz, & R. M. Jaffee (Eds.), *New concepts in gynecological oncology: A Hahnemann Symposium* (pp. 211 ff.). Philadelphia: F. A. Davis.

Gresham, M. L. (1976). The infantilization of the elderly: A developing concept. *Nursing Forum, 15,* 195–210.

Grove, R. D., & Hetzel, A. M. (1968). *Vital statistics rates in the United States, 1940-1960* (DHEW Publication No. PHS 1677). Washington, DC: U.S. Government Printing Office.

Gruenberg, E. M. (1977). The failures of success. *Millbank Memorial Fund Quarterly: Health and Society, 55,* 3–24.

Gubrium, J. F. (1975). *Living and dying at Murray Manor.* New York: St. Martin's.

Gurin, G., Veroff, J., & Field, F. (1960). *Americans view their mental health.* New York: Basic Books.

Gurland, B. J. (1976). The comparative frequency of depression in various adult age groups. *Journal of Gerontology, 31,* 283-292.

Gutman, G. M., Herbert, C. P., & Brown, S. R. (1977). Feldenkreis versus conventional exercises for the elderly. *Journal of Gerontology, 32,* 562-572.

Hacker, H. M. (1951). Women as a minority group. *Social Forces, 30,* 60-69.

Hagestad, G. O. (1982). Parent and child: Generations in the family. In T. M. Field, A. Huston, H. C. Quay, L. Troll, & G. E. Finley (Eds.), *Review of human development* (pp. 485-499). New York: Wiley.

Hagestad, G. O., & Kranichfeld, M. (1982, October). *Issues in the study of intergenerational continuity.* Paper presented at the NCFR Theory and Methods Workshop, Washington, DC.

Hagestad, G. O., Smyer, M. A., & Stierman, K. L. (1984). Parent-child relations in adulthood: The impact of divorce in middle age. In R. S. Cohen, B. J. Cohler, & S. Weissman (Eds.), *Parenthood: A psychodynamic perspective.* New York: Guilford.

Hamburg, D. A., Elliott, G. R., & Parron, D. L. (Eds.). (1982). *Health and behavior: Frontiers of research in the biobehavioral sciences.* Washington, DC: National Academy Press.

Hamilton, M. (1960). A rating scale for depression. *Journal of Neurology, Neurosurgery, and Psychiatry, 23,* 56-62.

Hamilton, M. (1967). Development of a rating scale for primary depressive illness. *British Journal of Social and Clinical Psychology, 6,* 278-296.

Hansard, S. L., Comar, C. L., & Plumlee, M. P. (1954). The effects of age upon calcium utilization and maintenance requirements in the bovine. *Journal of Animal Science, 13,* 25-36.

Harrison, G. G., & Fung, E. E. (1982). Nutritional therapy. In K. A. Conrad & R. Bressler (Eds.), *Drug therapy for the elderly* (pp. 91-111). St. Louis, MO: C. V. Mosby.

Harrison, J. E., McNeill, K. G., Sturtridge, W. C., Bayley, T. A., Murray, T. M., Williams, C., Tam, C., & Fornasier, V. (1981). Three-year changes in bone mineral mass of postmenopausal osteoporotic patients based on neutron activation analysis of the central third of the skeleton. *Journal of Clinical Endocrinology and Metabolism, 52,* 751-758.

Heaney, R. P. (1965). A unified concept of osteoporosis. *American Journal of Medicine, 39,* 887-880.

Heaney, R. P., Recker, R. R., & Saville, P. D. (1978). Menopausal changes in calcium balance performance. *Journal of Laboratory and Clinical Medicine, 92,* 953-963.

Hecox, B., Levine, E., & Scott, D. (1976). Dance in physical rehabilitation. *Physical Therapy, 56,* 919-924.

Hendricks, J., Hetzel, B., & Kahana, E. (1978, November). *Correlates of expanded and contracted social relationships in homes for the aged.* Paper presented at the 31st Annual Scientific Meeting of the Gerontological Society of America, Dallas, TX.

Henrard, J. C. (1980). Epidemiology of disablement in the elderly. *International Rehabilitation Medicine, 2*(4), 167–171.

Henry, J. (1963). *Culture against man.* New York: Random House.

Hess, B. B. (1979). Sex roles, friendship, and the life course. *Research on Aging, 1,* 494–515.

Hess, B. B., & Waring, J. M. (1978). Parent and child in later life: Rethinking the relationship. In R. M. Lerner & G. B. Spanier (Eds.), *Child influences on marital and family interaction: A life-span perspective* (pp. 241–273). New York: Academic.

Hill, R., Foote, N., Aldous, J., Carlson, R., & MacDonald, R. (1970). *Family development in three generations: A longitudinal study of changing family patterns of planning and achievement.* Cambridge, MA: Schenkman.

Hill, R. D. (1967). The prevalence of anemia in the over-65s in a rural practice. *Practitioner, 217,* 963–967.

Hillyard, C. J., Stevenson, J. C., & MacIntyre, I. (1978). Relative deficiency of plasma-calcitonin in normal women. *Lancet, i,* 961–962.

Hing, E. (1981). Characteristics of nursing home residents, health status, and care received: National Nursing Home Survey, United States, May-December 1977. *Vital and Health Statistics. Series 13,* NO. 51. (DHHS Publication No. PHS 81-1712). Washington, DC: U.S. Government Printing Office.

Hogue, C. C. (1982). Injury in late life: Part I. Epidemiology. *Journal of the American Geriatrics Society, 30,* 183–190.

Hollister, L. E. (1981). General principles of treating the elderly with drugs. In L. F. Jarvik, D. J. Greenblatt, & D. Harman (Eds.), *Aging, Vol. 16.* Clinical pharmacology and the aged patient (pp. 1–9). New York: Raven.

Horn, J. L., & Donaldson, G. (1980). Cognitive development in adulthood. In O. G. Brim & J. Kagan (Eds.), *Constancy and change in human development* (pp. 445–529). Cambridge MA: Harvard University Press.

Horsman, A., Gallagher, J. C., Simpson, M., & Nordin, B. E. C. (1977). Prospective trial of oestrogen and calcium in postmenopausal women. *British Medical Journal, 2,* 789–792.

Hrdy, S. B. (1981). *The woman that never evolved.* Cambridge, MA: Harvard University Press.

Hughes, G. (1969). Changes in taste sensitivity with advancing age. *Gerontologia Clinica, 11,* 224–230.

Hunt, K. E., Fry, D. E., & Bland, K. I. (1980). Breast carcinoma in the elderly patient: An assessment of operative risk, morbidity, and mortality. *American Journal of Surgery, 140,* 339–342.

Hunt, T. E., (1980). Practical considerations in the rehabilitation of the aged. *Journal of the American Geriatrics Society, 28,* 59–64.

Hurvitz, M. (1969). Predisposing factors in adverse reactions to drugs. *British Medical Journal 1,* 536–539.

Hutchinson, T. A., Polansky, S. M., & Feinstein, A. R. (1979). Post-menopausal oestrogens protect against fractures of hip and distal radius: A case-control study. *Lancet, ii*, 705–709.

Ingbar, S. H. (1978). Influence of aging on the human thyroid hormone economy. In R. B. Greenblatt (Ed.), *Aging* (Vol. 5). *Geriatric endocrinology* (pp. 13ff.). New York: Raven.

ISR Newsletter. (1977, Winter). Ann Arbor, MI: University of Michigan, Institute of Social Research.

Jackson, J. (1967). Social gerontology and the negro: A review. *Gerontologist, 7*, 167–178.

Jackson, J. *Quadruple jeopardy: Being old and black and female and poor.* (1971). Paper presented at the 24th Annual Meeting of the Gerontological Society of America, Houston, TX.

Jackson, J. (1982). Death rates of aged blacks and whites, United States, 1964–1978. *The Black Scholar, 13*, 36–48.

Jackson, J., & Walls, B. E. (1978). Myths and realities about aged blacks. In. M. R. Brown (Ed.), *Readings in gerontology* (2nd ed., pp. 95–113). St. Louis: C. V. Mosby.

Jackson, M., Kolody, B., & Wood, J. L. (1982). To be old and black: The case for double jeopardy on income and health. In R. C. Manuel (Ed.), *Minority aging: Sociological and social psychological issues* (pp. 77–82). Westport, CT: Greenwood.

Jackson, M., & Wood, J. L. (1976). *Implications for the black aged.* Washington, DC: National Council on Aging.

Jette, A. M., & Branch, L. G. (1981). The Framingham Disability Study: II. Physical disability among the aging. *American Journal of Public Health, 71*, 1211–1216.

Jick, H., Slone, D., Borda, I. T., & Shapiro, S. (1968). Efficacy and toxicity of heparin in relation to age and sex. *New England Journal of Medicine, 279*, 284–286.

Johnson, C. L., & Catalano, D. J. (1981). Childless elderly and their family supports. *Gerontologist, 21*, 610–618.

Jordan, V. B. (1980). Conserving kinship concepts: A developmental study in social cognition. *Child Developmen, 51*, 146–155.

Judd, H. L., Judd, G. E., Lucas, W. E., & Yeh, S. S. (1974). Endocrine function of the postmenopausal ovary: Concentration of androgens and estrogens in ovarian and peripheral vein blood. *Journal of Clinical Endocrinology and Metabolism, 39*, 1020–1024.

Judd, H. L., Lucas, W. E., & Yeh, S. S. C. (1976). Serum 17-beta-estradiol and estrone levels in postmenopausal women with and without endometrial cancer. *Journal of Clinical Endocrinology and Metabolism, 43*, 272–278.

Kahana, B. (1975, June). *Competent coping: A psychotherapeutic strategy.* Paper presented at the International Gerontological Association, Jerusalem.

Kahana, B. (1982). Social behavior and aging. In B. Wolman & G. Stricker (Eds.), *Handbook of developmental psychology* (pp. 871–889). Englewood Cliffs, NJ: Prentice-Hall.

Kahana, B., & Kahana, E. (1979, August). *Strategies of coping in institutional environments.* Final Progress Report, NIH Grant No. 24959-04. Bethesda, MD: National Institutes of Health.

Kahana, E. (1973). The humane treatment of old people in institutions. *Gerontologist, 13,*(3, Pt. 1), 282–289.

Kahana, E. (1975, January). *Service needs of the urban aged: Perspectives of consumers, agencies, and significant others.* Paper presented at the Pro-Seminar of the Wayne-State University–University of Michigan Institute of Gerontology.

Kahana, E., & Coe, R. M. (1969). Dimensions of conformity: A multidisciplinary view. *Journal of Gerontology, 24,* 76–81.

Kahana, E., & Kiyak, H. A. (1980). The older woman: Impact of widowhood and living arrangements on service needs. *Journal of Gerontological Social Work, 3,* 17–29.

Kahana, E., & Kiyak, H. A. (1982, November). *Observing staff-client interactions in facilities for the aged.* Paper presented at the 35th Annual Scientific Meeting of the Gerontological Society of America, Boston.

Kahana, E., & Kiyak, H. A. (1983, November). *A multidimensional concept of attitudes toward the elderly: Its measurement and antecedents.* Paper presented in the Symposium on Behavioral Geriatrics Research, 36th Annual Scientific Meeting of the Gerontological Society of America, San Francisco.

Kahana, E., Liang, J., & Felton, B. J. (1980). Alternative models of person-environment fit: Prediction of morale in three homes for the aged. *Journal of Gerontology, 35,* 584–595.

Kahn, R. L. (1981). *Work and health.* New York: Wiley.

Kallman, K. D. (1962). Population genetics of the gynogenetic teleost. *Mollienesia formosa* (Girard). *Evolution, 16,* 497–504.

Kamath, S. K. (1982). Taste acuity and aging. *American Journal of Clinical Nutrition, 36,* 766–775.

Kane, R., Solomon, D., Beck, J., Keeler, E., & Kane, R. (1980). The future need for geriatric manpower in the United States. *New England Journal of Medicine, 302,* 1327–1332.

Kane, R. L., Solomon, D. H., Beck, J. C., Keeler, E., & Kane, R. A. (1980). *Geriatrics in the United States: Manpower projections and training considerations.* Santa Monica, CA: The Rand Corporation.

Karmody, A. M., & Leather, R. P. (1979). Guidelines for vascular surgery referral. *Geriatrics, 34,* 45–54.

Kart, C. (1981). Experiencing symptoms: Attribution and misattribution of illness among the aged. In M. R. Haug (Ed.), *Elderly patients and their doctors* (pp. 70–78). New York: Springer.

Kart, C. S., & Manard, B. B.(1976). Quality of care in old age institutions. *Gerontologist, 16,* 250–256.

Kasl, S. V. (1972). Physical and mental health effects of involuntary relocation and institutionalization of the elderly—A review. *American Journal of Public Health, 62,* 377–384.

Katz, B. P., Zdeb, M. S., and Therriault, G. D. (1979). Where people die. *Public Health Reports, 94,* 522–527.

Keyfitz, N. (1977). What difference would it make if cancer were eradicated? An examination of the Taeuber Paradox. *Demography, 14,* 411–418.

Keyfitz, N. (1978). Improving life expectancy: An uphill road ahead. *American Journal of Public Health, 68,* 954–956.

Kiesler, S. B., & Shanas, E. (Eds.). (1981). *Aging: Stability and change in the family* (pp. 47–81). New York: Academic.

Kish, L. (1965). *Survey sampling.* New York: Wiley.

Klaiber, E. L., Broverman, D. M., Vogel, W., & Kobayashi, Y. (1979). Estrogen therapy for severe persistent depressions in women. *Archives of General Psychiatry, 36,* 550–554.

Knowles, J. H. (1977). The responsibility of the individual. *Daedalus, Winter,* 57–80.

Kogan, N. (1979). A study of age categorization. *Journal of Gerontology, 34,* 358–367.

Koger, L. J. (1980). Nursing home life satisfaction and activity participation: Effect of a resident-written magazine. *Research on Aging, 2,* 61–72.

Kohn, M. L. (1981). Personality, occupation, and social stratification: A frame of reference. In D. J. Treiman & R. V. Robinson (Eds.), *Research on social stratification and mobility* (Vol. 1, pp. 267–297). Greenwich, CT: JAI.

Kosberg, J. I., & Tobin, S. S. (1972). Variability among nursing homes. *Gerontologist, 12,* 214–219.

Kottke, F. J. (1966). The effects of limitation of activity upon the human body. *Journal of the American Medical Association, 196*(10), 825–830.

Kreiger, N., Kelsey, J. L., Holford, T. R., & O'Connor, T. (1982). An epidemiological study of hip fracture in postmenopausal women. *American Journal of Epidemiology, 116,* 141–148.

Ladosky, W., & Gazeri, L. C. (1979). Brain serotonin and sexual differentiation of the nervous system. *Neuroendocrinology, 6,* 168–174.

Lamy, P. P. (1982). Comparative pharmacokinetic changes and drug therapy in an older population. *Journal of the American Geriatrics Society, 30* (Suppl.), S11–S19.

Langer, E., & Rodin, J. (1976). The effects of choice and enhanced personal responsibility: A field experiment in institutional setting. *Journal of Personality and Social Psychology, 34,* 191–198.

Lauritzen, C. (1973). The management of the pre-menopausal and the postmenopausal patient. In P. A. van Keep & C. Lauritzen (Eds.), *Frontiers in hormone research,* Vol. 2 (pp. 2–21). Basel: S. Karger.

Lawton, M. P. (1970). Public behavior of older people in congregate housing. In J. Archea & C. Eastmen (Eds.), *Environmental Design Research Association II.* Pittsburgh: Carnegie-Mellon University.

Lawton, M. P., & Nahemow, L. E. (1973). Ecology and the aging process. In C. Eisdorfer & M. P. Lawton (Eds.), *Psychology of adult development and aging* (pp. 619–674). Washington, DC: American Psychological Association.

Learoyd, B. M. (1972). Psychotropic drugs in the elderly. *Medical Journal of Australia, 1,* (22) 1131–1133.

Lehr, U. (1982). Hat die Grossfamilie heute noch eine Chance? *Der Deutsche Arzt 18,* Sonderdruck.

Lehr, U. (1983, February). *The role of women in the family generation context.* International Symposium on Intergenerational Relationships, Berlin.

Leichter, H. J., & Mitchell, W. E. (1973). *Kinship and casework: Family networks and social interactions.* New York: Russell Sage Foundation.

Lesser, M. (1978). The effects of rhythmic exercise on the range of motion in older adults. *American Corrective Therapy Journal, 32,* 118–122.

Levey, S., Ruchlin, H. S., Stotsky, B. A., Kinlock, D. R., & Oppenheim, W. (1973). An appraisal of nursing home care. *Journal of Gerontology, 28,* 222–228.

Lewis, A. F. (1981). Fracture of neck of femur: Changing incidence. *British Medical Journal, 283,* 1217–1220.

Lewis, R. (1976). Anemia—a common but never a concomitant of aging. *Geriatrics, 31,* 53–60.

Lieberman, G. L. (in press). Children of the elderly as natural helpers: Some demographic variables. In J. C. Glidewell & M. A. Lieberman (Spec. Issue Eds.), *American Journal of Community Psychology.*

Lieberman, M. A. (1969). Institutionalization of the aged: Effects on behavior. *Journal of Gerontology, 24,* 330–340.

Lieberman, M. A., & Lakin, M. (1963). On becoming an institutionalized person. In R. M. Williams, C. Tibbits, & W. Donahue (Eds.), *Process of aging* (Vol. I). *Social and psychological perspectives* (pp. 475–503). New York: Atherton.

Liljestrom, R. (1971). On vertical differentiation of sex roles: Age classes among the Myakusa and patterns of interaction in Swedish children's books. *Acta Sociologica, 14,* 13–23.

Lindemann, E. (1944). Symptomatology and management of acute grief. *American Journal of Psychiatry, 101,* 141–148.

Lindsay, R., & Hart, D. M. (1978). Oestrogens and postmenopausal bone loss. *Scottish Medical Journal, 23,* 13–18.

Lindsay, R., & Hart, D. M. (1982). Unpublished raw data.

Lindsay, R., Hart, D. M., Aitken, J. M., MacDonald, E. B., Anderson, J. B., & Clark, A. (1976). Long-term prevention of postmenopausal osteoporosis by oestrogens. *Lancet, ii,* 1038–1040.

Lindsay, R., Hart, D. M., Forrest, C., & Baird, C. (1980). Prevention of spinal osteoporosis in oophorectomized women. *Lancet, ii*, 1151–1153.

Lindsay, R., Hart, D. M., & Kraszewski, A. (1980). Prospective double-blind trial of synthetic steroid (ORG OD 14) for preventing postmenopausal osteoporosis. *British Medical Journal, 280*, 1207–1209.

Lindsay, R., Hart, D. M., MacLean, A., Clark, A. C., Kraszewski, A., & Garwood, J. (1978). Bone response to termination of oestrogen treatment. *Lancet, i*, 1325–1327.

Lindsay, R., Hart, D. M., Purdie, D., Ferguson, M. M., Clark, A. S., & Kraszewski, A. (1978). Comparative effects of estrogen and a progestogen on bone loss in postmenopausal women. *Clinical Science and Molecular Medicine, 54*, 193–195.

Lindsay, R., & Herrington, B. S. (In preparation). Osteoporotic fractures in the U.S.A.

Linn, B. S., Linn, M. W., & Wallen, N. (1982). Evaluation of results in surgical procedures in the elderly. *Annals of Surgery, 195*, 90–96.

Lipschitz, D. A. (1982). Protein calorie malnutrition in the hospitalized elderly. *Primary Care, 9*, 531–543.

Lipschitz, D. A., & Mitchell, C. O. (1980). Enteral hyperalimentation and hematopoietic toxicity caused by chemotherapy of small cell lung cancer. *Journal of Parenteral and Enteral Nutrition, 4*, 583.

Lipschitz, D. A., & Mitchell, C. O. (1982). The correctability of the nutritional, immune, and hematopoietic manifestations of protein calorie malnutrition in the elderly. *Journal of the American College of Nutrition, 1*, 17–25.

Lipschitz, D. A., Mitchell, C. O., & Thomson, C. (1981). The anemia of senescence. *American Journal of Hematology, 11*, 47–54.

Livson, F. B. (1976). Patterns of personality development in middle-aged women: A longitudinal study. *International Journal of Aging and Human Development, 7*, 107–115.

Loether, H. J. (1975). *Problems of aging: Sociological and social psychological perspectives* (2nd ed.). Encino, CA: Dickinson.

Lopata, H. Z. (1971). Widows as a minority group. *Gerontologist, 11*, 67–77.

Lopata, H. Z. (1973). *Widowhood in an American city*. Cambridge, MA: Schenkman.

Lopata, H. Z. (1975). Grief work and identity reconstruction. *Journal of Geriatric Psychiatry, 8*, 41–55.

Lopata, H. Z. (1979). *Women as widows: Support systems*. New York: Elsevier.

Lorber, J. (1981). *Questioning assumptions about disabled women: A look at chronic renal failure patients*. Paper presented at the Annual Meeting of the Society for the Study of Social Problems, Toronto, Canada.

Lovejoy, C. O. (1981). The origin of man. *Science, 211*, 341–350.

Lowenthal, M., & Robinson, B. (1976). Social networks and isolation. In

R. Binstock & E. Shanas (Eds.), *Handbook of aging and the social sciences* (pp. 432–456). New York: Van Nostrand Reinhold.

Lutwak, L., Krook, L., Henrikson, P. A., Uris, R., Whalen, J., Coulston, A., & Lesser, G. (1971). Calcium deficiency and human periodontal disease. *Israel Journal of Medical Science, 7,* 504–509.

Mace, N. S., & Rabins, P. V. (1981). *The 36-hour-day: A family guide to caring for persons with Alzheimer's disease, related dementing illnesses and memory loss in later life.* Baltimore: Johns Hopkins University Press.

MacLennan, W. J., Martin, P., & Mason, B. J. (1977). Protein intake and serum albumin levels in the elderly. *Gerontology, 23,* 360–367.

Maddison, D., & Viola, A. (1968). The health of widows in the year following bereavement. *Journal of Psychosomatic Research, 12,* 297–306.

Manton, K. G. (1980). Sex and race specific mortality in multiple cause of death data. *Gerontologist, 20,* 480–493.

Manton, K. G. (1982). Changing concepts of morbidity and mortality in the elderly populations. *Milbank Memorial Fund Quarterly: Health and Society, 60,* 183–244.

Manton, K. G., Poss, S. S., & Wing, S. (1979). The black-white mortality crossover: Investigation from the perspective of the components of aging. *Gerontologist, 19,* 291–300.

Margulec, I., Librach, G., & Schadel, M. (1970). Epidemiological study of accidents among residents of homes for the aged. *Journal of Gerontology, 25,* 342–346.

Marshall, V. W., Rosenthal, C. J., & Synge, J. (1983). Concerns about parental health. In E. M. Markson (Ed.), *Older women: Issues and prospects* (pp. 253–274). Lexington, MA: Lexington.

Martinez, R. L., & Kidd, A. H. (1980). Two personality characteristics in adult pet-owners and non-owners. *Psychological Reports, 47,* 318.

Martkovic, V., Kostial, K., Simonovic, I., Buzina, R., Brodarec, A., & Nordin, B. E. C. (1979). Bone status and fracture rates in two regions of Yugoslavia. *American Journal of Clinical Nutrition, 32,* 540–549.

Maurer, K. (1979). Basic data on arthritis: Knee, hip, and sacroiliac joints, in adult ages 25–74 years, United States, 1971–1975. *Vital and Health Statistics. Series 11,* No. 213 (DHEW Publication No. PHS 79-1661). Washington, DC: U.S. Government Printing Office.

McConnel, C. E., & Deljavan, F. (1982). Aged deaths: The nursing home community differential, 1976. *Gerontologist, 22,* 314–317.

McWhorter, J. M. (1980). Group therapy for high utilizers of clinic facilities. In I. M. Burnside (Ed.), *Psychosocial nursing care of the aged* (2nd ed., pp. 114–125). New York: McGraw-Hill.

Mendelson, M. A. (1974). *Tender loving greed—How the incredibly lucrative nursing home "industry" is exploiting America's old people and defrauding us all.* New York: Alfred K. Knopf.

Metropolitan Life Foundation. (1982). Health of the elderly. *Statistical Bulletin, 63,* 2–5.

Meyerson, M. D. (1976). The effects of aging on communication. *Journal of Gerontology, 31,* 29–38.

Migeon, C. J., Keller, A. R., Lawrence, B., & Shepard, T. H. (1957). Dehydro-epiandroseterone and androsterone levels in human plasma. Effect of age and sex: day-to-day and diurnal variations. *Journal of Clinical Endocrinology, 17,* 1051–1062.

Miller, C., & LeLieuvre, R. B. (1982). A method to reduce chronic pain in elderly nursing home residents. *Gerontologist, 22,* 314–317.

Milleren, J. W. (1977). Some contingencies affecting the utilization of tranquilizers in long-term care of the elderly. *Journal of Health and Social Behavior, 18,* 206–211.

Mitchell, C. O., & Lipschitz, D. A. (1982a). Detection of protein calorie malnutrition in the elderly. *American Journal of Clinical Nutrition, 35,* 398–406.

Mitchell, C. O., & Lipschitz, D. A. (1982b). The effect of age and sex on the routinely used measurements to assess the nutritional status of hospitalized patients. *American Journal of Clinical Nutrition, 36,* 340–349.

Moaz, B., & Durst, N. (1979). Psychology of the menopause. In P. A. van Keep, D. M. Serr, R. B. Greenblatt (Eds.), *Female and male climacteric: Current opinion 1978* (pp. 9ff.). Lancaster, England: MTP Press.

Moore, J. T. (1978). Functional disability of geriatric patients in a family medicine program: Implications for patient care, education, and research. *Journal of Family Practice, 7,* 1159–1166.

Morgan, L. A. (1976). A re-examination of widowhood and morale. *Journal of Gerontology, 31,* 687–695.

Morgan, L. A. (1980). Work in widowhood: A viable option? *Gerontologist, 20,* 581–587.

Morris, J. M. (1961). Functional tumors of the ovary. *Clinical Obstetrics and Gynecology, 4,* 821–833.

Morris, S. (1972). *Grief and how to live with it.* New York: Grosset & Dunlap.

Mossey, J. M., & Shapiro, E. (1982). Self-rated health: A predictor of mortality among the elderly. *American Journal of Public Health, 72,* 800–808.

Myers, M. A., Saunders, C. R. G., & Chalmers, D. G. (1968). The hemoglobin level of fit elderly people. *Lancet, ii,* 261–263.

Nachtigall, L. E., Nachtigall, R. H., Nachtigall, R. D., & Beckman, E. M. (1979). Estrogen replacement therapy. I: A 10-year prospective study in the relationship to osteoporosis. *Obstetrics and Gynecology, 53,* 277–281.

Nagi, S. Z. (1976). An epidemiology of disability among adults in the United States. *Milbank Memorial Fund Quarterly: Health and Society, 54,* 439–467.

Nam, C. B., Weatherby, N. L., & Ockay, K. A. (1978). Causes of death which contribute to the mortality crossover effect. *Social Biology, 25,* 306–314.

Nation, R. L., Triggs, E. J., & Selig, M. (1976). Lignocaine kinetics in cardiac patients and aged subjects. *British Journal of Clinical Pharmacology, 3,* 327–367.

National Cancer Institute. (1981). Surveillance, epidemiology, and end results: Incidence and mortality data, 1973–77. *National Cancer Institute Monographs, No. 57* (NIH Publication No. 81-23300). Washington, DC: U.S. Government Printing Office.

National Center for Health Statistics (1974). *Vital and Health Statistics, Series 10,* No. 96. Washington, DC: U.S. Government Printing Office.

National Center for Health Statistics. (1977). *Vital and Health Statistics, Series, 11,* No. 201. Washington, DC: U.S. Government Printing Office.

National Center for Health Statistics. (1978a). *Health. United States, 1978* (DHEW Publication No. PHS 78-1232). Washington, DC: U.S. Government Printing Office.

National Center for Health Statistics. (1978b). *Vital and Health Statistics, Series 10,* No. 126. Washington, DC: U.S. Government Printing Office.

National Center for Health Statistics. (1978c). *Vital and Health Statistics, Series 11,* No. 205. Washington, DC: U.S. Government Printing Office.

National Center for Health Statistics. (1978d). *Vital and Health Statistics, Series 11,* No. 212. Washington, DC: U.S. Government Printing Office.

National Center for Health Statistics. (1978e). *Vital and Health Statistics, Series 13,* No. 33, Washington, DC: U.S. Government Printing Office.

National Center for Health Statistics. (1978f). *Vital and Health Statistics, Series 13,* No. 35. Washington, DC: U.S. Government Printing Office.

National Center for Health Statistics. (1979a). *Health. United States, 1978* (DHHS Publication No. 78-12321-1). Washington, DC: U.S. Government Printing Office.

National Center for Health Statistics (1979b). *Vital and Health Statistics, Series 10,* No. 130. Washington, DC: U.S. Government Printing Office.

National Center for Health Statistics. (1979c). *Vital and Health Statistics, Series 11,* No. 213. Washington, DC: U.S. Government Printing Office.

National Center for Health Statistics. (1979d). *Vital and Health Statistics, Series 11,* No. 214. Washington, DC: U.S. Government Printing Office.

National Center for Health Statistics. (1980a). Advance report, final mortality statistics, 1978. *Monthly Vital Statistics Report, 29,* No. 6 (Suppl. 2), September 17. Washington, DC: U.S. Government Printing Office.

National Center for Health Statistics. (1980b). *Health. United States, 1980* (DHHS Publication No. PHS 81-1232). Washington, DC: U.S. Government Printing Office.

National Center for Health Statistics. (1980c). *Vital and Health Statistics, Series 11,* No. 215. Washington, DC: U.S. Government Printing Office.

National Center for Health Statistics. (1981a). *Vital and Health Statistics, Series 11,* No. 221. Washington, DC: U.S. Government Printing Office.

National Center for Health Statistics. (1981b). *Vital and Health Statistics, Series 13,* No. 59. Washington, DC: U.S. Government Printing Office.

National Center for Health Statistics Research. (1967). *Eighth revision International Classification of Diseases.* (U.S. Publication No. PHS 1693). Washington, DC: Author.

National Council on the Aging, Inc. (1976). *The myth and reality of aging in America.* Washington, DC: Author.

National Institute of Mental Health. (1977). *Research on the mental health of the aging 1960-1976.* (DHEW Publication No. ADM 77-379). Rockville, MD: Author.

National Research Council. Committee on Dietary Allowances. (1980). *Recommended dietary allowances* (9th ed.). Washington, DC: National Academy of Sciences.

National Urban League. (1964). *Double jeopardy: The older negro in America today.* New York: Author.

Neugarten, B. L. (1968). The awareness of middle age. In B. L. Neugarten (Ed.), *Middle age and aging* (pp. 93–98). Chicago: University of Chicago Press. (Reprinted from R. Owen [Ed.]. [1967]. *Middle age and aging.* London: British Broadcasting Corporation.)

Neugarten, B. L. (1979). The middle generations. In P. K. Ragan (Ed.), *Aging parents* (pp. 258–266), Monograph, the Ethel Percy Andrus Foundation. Los Angeles: University of Southern California Press.

Neugarten, B. L., & Datan, N. (1973). Sociological perspectives on the life-cycle. In P. Baltes & K. W. Schaie (Eds.), *Life-span developmental psychology: Personality and socialization* (pp. 53–69). New York: Academic.

Neugarten, B. L., & Guttman, D. (1964). Age-sex roles and personality in middle age: A thematic apperception study. In B. L. Neugarten (Ed.), *Personality in middle and later life: Empirical studies* (pp. 44–89). New York: Atherton.

Neugarten, B. L., Wood, V., Kraines, R. J., & Loomis, B. (1963). Women's attitudes toward the menopause. *Vita Humana, 6,* 141–151.

Nockerts, S. R., Detmer, D. E., & Fryback, D. G. (1980). Incidental appendectomy in the elderly? No. *Surgery, 8,* 301–306.

Novak, L. P. (1972). Aging, total body potassium, fat-free mass and cell mass in males and females between ages 18 and 85 years. *Journal of Gerontology, 27,* 438–443.

Oddie, T. H., Myhill, J., Pirnique, F. G., & Fisher, D. A. (1968). Effect of age and sex on the radio-iodine uptake in euthyroid subjects. *Journal of Clinical Endocrinology and Metabolism, 28,* 776–782.

O'Donnell, T. F., Jr., Darling, R. C., & Linton, R. R. (1976). Is 80 years too old for aneurysmectomy? *Archives of Surgery, 111,* 1250–1257.

Oppenheimer, V. K. (1981). The changing nature of life-cycle squeezes: Implications for the socio-economic position of the elderly. In R. W. Fogel, E. Hatfield, S. B. Kiesler (Eds.), *Aging: Stability and change in the family* (pp. 47–81). New York: Academic.

Ouslander, J. G. (1981). Drug therapy in the elderly. *Annals of Internal Medicine, 95,* 711-722.

Pablo, R. Y. (1977). Patient accidents in a long-term care facility. *Canadian Journal of Public Health, 63,* 237-247.

Pak, C. Y. C., Stewart, A., Kaplan, R., Bone, H., Notz, C., & Browne, R. (1975). Photon absorptiometric analysis of bone density in primary hyperparathyroidism. *Lancet, ii,* 7-8.

Palmore, E. B. (1969a). Physical, mental, and social factors in predicting longevity. *Gerontologist, 9,* 103-108.

Palmore, E. B. (1969b). Predicting longevity: A follow-up controlling for age. *Gerontologist, 9,* 247-250.

Palmore, E. B. (1976). Total chance of institutionalization among the aged. *Gerontologist, 16,* 504-507.

Palmore, E. B., & Luikart, C. (1972). Health and social factors related to life satisfaction. *Journal of Health and Social Behavior, 13,* 68-80.

Parkes, C. M. (1972). *Bereavement: Studies of grief in adult life.* New York: International Universities Press.

Parsons, J. A., Meunier, P. J., Neer, R. M., Podbesek, R., & Reeve, J. (1981). Effects of synthetic human parathyroid hormone fragment (hPTH 1-34) on bone mass and bone mineral metabolism. In H. F. DeLuca, H. M. Frost, W. S. S. Jee, C. C. Johnston, Jr., & A. M. Parfitt (Eds.), *Osteoporosis: Recent advances in pathogenesis and treatment: Proceedings of the 10th Steenbock Symposium* (pp. 457-465). Baltimore: University Park Press.

Parsons, T., & Bales, R. F. (1955). *Family, socialization, and interaction process.* New York: The Free Press.

Payne, B. P., & Whittington, F. (1976). Older women: Examination of popular stereotypes and research evidence. *Social Problems, 23,* 288-504.

Pearlin, L. I., & Schooler, C. (1978). The structure of coping. *Journal of Health and Social Behavior, 19,* 2-21.

Penfield, W. (1968). In M. B. Strauss (Ed.), *Familiar medical quotations.* Boston: Little Brown.

Perlmutter, M. (1983). Learning and memory through adulthood. In M. W. Riley, B. B. Hess, & K. Bond (Eds.), *Aging in society: Selected reviews of recent research* (pp. 219). Hillsdale, NJ: L. Erlbaum.

Peters, L. (1982). Women's health care. Approaches in delivery to physically disabled women. *Nurse Practitioner, 7,* 34-37, 48.

Petracek, M. R., & Lawson, J. D., Rhea, W. G., Jr., Ritchie, R. E., & Dean, R. H. (1980). Resection of abdominal aortic aneurysms in the over-80 age group. *Southern Medical Journal, 73,* 579-581.

Pfeiffer, E. (1970). Survival in old age: Physical, psychological, and social correlates of longevity. *Journal of the American Geriatrics Society, 28,* 273-285.

Phillips, L. R. F. (1980). *Family relationships between two samples of frail elderly individuals.* Unpublished doctoral dissertation, University of Arizona.

Poon, L. W., Walsh-Sweeney, L., & Fozard, J. L. (1980). Memory skill training for the elderly: Salient issues on the use of imagery mnemonics. In L. W. Poon, J. L. Fozard, L. S. Cermak, D. Arenberg, & L. W. Thompson, *New directions in memory and aging: Proceedings of the George A. Talland Memorial Conference* (pp. 461–484). Hillsdale, NJ: L. Erlbaum.

Poortman, J., Thijssen, J. H. H., & Schwarz, F. (1973). Androgen production and conversion to estrogens in normal postmenopausal women and in selected breast cancer patients. *Journal of Clinical Endocrinology and Metabolism, 37,* 101–109.

Powers, J. H. (Ed.) (1968). *Surgery of the aged and debilitated patient.* Philadelphia: W. B. Saunders.

Preston, S. H. (1976). Family sizes of children and family sizes of women. *Demography, 13,* 105–114.

Procopé, B. J. (1968). Studies of the urinary excretion, biological effects and origin of oestrogens in postmenopausal women. *Acta Endocrinologica, 60* (Suppl. 135).

Public Health Service. (1959). Limitation of activity and mobility due to chronic conditions, United States, July 1957–June 1958. *Health Statistics. Series B, No. 11.* Washington, DC.

Rader, M. D., Flickinger, G. L., de Villa, G. O., Mikuta, J. J., & Mikhail, G. (1973). Plasma estrogens in postmenopausal women. *American Journal of Obstetrics and Gynecology, 116,* 1069–1073.

Radloff, L. S. (1977). The CES-D Scale: A self-report depression scale for research in the general population. *Applied Psychological Measurement, 1,* 385–401.

Raskin, A., & Jarvik, L. F. (Eds.). (1979). *Psychiatric symptoms and cognitive loss in the elderly: Evaluation and assessment techniques.* New York: Wiley.

Recker, R. R., Saville, P. D., & Heaney, R. P. (1977). Effect of estrogens and calcium carbonate on bone loss in postmenopausal women. *Annals of Internal Medicine, 87,* 649–655.

Rees, W. D. (1971). The hallucinations of widowhood. *British Medical Journal, 4,* 37–41.

Reiss, P. J. (1962). The extended kinship system: Correlates of and attitudes on frequency of interaction. *Marriage and Family Living, 24,* 333–339.

Ridley, J. C., Bachrach, C. A., & Dawson, D. A. (1979). Recall and reliability of interview data from older women. *Journal of Gerontology, 34,* 99–105.

Riggs, B. L., Seeman, E., Hodgson, S. F., Taves, D. R., & O'Fallon, W. M. (1982). Effect of the fluoride/calcium regimen on vertebral fracture occurrence in postmenopausal osteoporosis. *New England Journal of Medicine, 306,* 446–450.

Riley, M. W. (1978). Aging, social change, and the power of ideas. *Daedalus, 107,* 39–52.

Riley, M. W. (1980). Age and aging: From theory generation to theory testing. In H. M. Blalock, Jr. (Ed.), *Sociological theory and research: A critical appraisal* (pp. 339–349). New York: The Free Press.

Riley, M. W. (1981a) Health behavior of older people: Toward a new paradigm. In D. L. Parron, F. Solomon, & J. Rodin (Eds.), *Health, behavior, and aging: Summary of a conference* (pp. 25–39). Washington, DC: National Academy Press.

Riley, M. W. (1981b). The healthy woman in the year 2000. In *Health issues of older women: A projection to the year 2000: Conference proceedings* (pp. 65–69). (Available from the School of Allied Health Professions, State University of New York at Stony Brook, Stony Brook, NY 11794.)

Riley, M. W. (1982). Implications for the middle and later years. In P. W. Berman & E. R. Ramey (Eds.), *Women: A developmental perspective* (pp. 399–405) (DHHS Publication No. PHS 82-2298). Washington, DC: U.S. Government Printing Office.

Riley, M. W., & Bond, K. (1983). Beyond ageism: Postponing the onset of disability. In M. W. Riley, B. B. Hess, & K. Bond (Eds.), *Aging in society: Selected reviews of recent research* (pp. 243–252). Hillsdale, NJ: L. Erlbaum.

Riley, M. W., & Foner, A. (1968). *Aging and society I: An inventory of research findings.* New York: Russell Sage Foundation.

Robins, L. N., Helzer, J. E., Croughan, J., & Ratcliffe, K. S. (1981). National Institute of Mental Health Diagnostic Interview Schedule: Its history, characteristics and validity. *Archives of General Psychiatry, 38,* 381–389.

Robinson, B., & Thurnher, M. (1979). Taking care of aged parents: A family cycle transition. *Gerontologist, 19,* 586–593.

Robson, K. S. (1974). Clinical report: Letters to a dead husband. *Journal of Geriatric Psychiatry, 7,* 208–232.

Rodin, J. (1980). Managing the stress of aging: The role of control and coping. In S. Levine & H. Ursin (Eds.), *Coping and health* (pp. 171–202). New York: Plenum.

Rogers, D. E., Blendon, R. J., & Moloney, T. W. (1982). Who needs Medicare? *New England Journal of Medicine, 307,* 13–18.

Rosen, J. L., & Neugarten, B. L. (1964). Ego functions in the middle and later years: A thematic apperception study. In B. L. Neugarten (Ed.), *Personality in middle and later life: Empirical studies* (pp. 90–101). New York: Atherton.

Rosenthal, C. J. (1981, November). *Kinkeeping: A task in the familial division of labor.* Paper presented at the combined 34th Annual Scientific Meeting of the Gerontological Society of America and the 10th Annual Meeting of the Canadian Association of Gerontology, Toronto, Canada. *Gerontologist, 21* (Spec. Issue), 306 [Abstr.].

Rosenwaike, I., Yaffe, N., & Sagi, C. (1980). The recent decline in mortality of the extreme aged: An analysis of statistical data. *American Journal of Public Health, 70,* 1074–1080.

Rosow, I. (1967). *The social integration of the aged.* New York: Free Press.

Roth, J., Glick, S. M., Yalow, R. S., & Berson, S. A. (1963). Hypoglycemia: A potent stimulus to secretion of growth hormone. *Science, 140,* 987–988.

Rowland, K. F. (1977). Environmental events predicting death for the elderly, *Psychological Bulletin, 84,* 349–372.

Ryder, N. B. (1964). Notes on the concept of a population, *American Journal of Sociology, 69,* 447–463.

Sandburg, C. (1970). The complete poems of Carl Sandburg. New York: Harcourt Brace Jovanovich.

Schaie, K. W., & Geiwitz, J. (1982). *Adult development and aging.* Boston: Little Brown.

Schaie, K. W., Orchowsky, S., & Parham, I. (1982). Measuring age and sociocultural change: The case of race and life satisfaction. In R. C. Manuel (Ed.), *Minority aging: Social and social psychological issues* (pp. 223–230).

Schiffman, S. S., Moss, J., & Erickson, R. P. (1976). Thresholds of food odors in the elderly. *Experimental Aging Research, 2,* 387–398.

Schultz, R., & Brenner, G. (1977). Relocation of the aged: Review and theoretical analysis. *Gerontologist, 32,* 323–333.

Schuman, J. E., Beattie, E. J., Steed, D. A., Merry, G. M., & Kraus, A. S. (1981). Geriatric patients with and without intellectual dysfunction: Effectiveness of a standard rehabilitation program. *Archives of Physical Medicine and Rehabilitation, 62,* 612–617.

Schwartz, A. N. (1979). Psychological dependency: An emphasis on the later years. In P. K. Ragan (Ed.) *Aging parents* (pp. 116–125). Ethel Percy Andrus Gerontology Center Monograph. Los Angeles: The University of Southern California.

Scott-Maxwell, F. (1968). *The measure of my days.* New York: Knopf.

Seidel, L. G., Thorton, G. F., Smith, J. W., & Cluff, L. E. (1966). Studies on the epidemiology of adverse drug reactions. III. Reactions in patients on a general medical service. *Bulletin of the Johns Hopkins Hospital, 119,* 229–315.

Shanas, E. (1962). *The health of older people: A social survey.* Cambridge, MA: Harvard University Press.

Shanas, E. (1979). Social myth as hypothesis: The case of the family relations of old people. *Gerontologist, 19,* 3–9.

Shanas, E. (1980). Older people and their families: The new pioneers. *Journal of Marriage and the Family, 42,* 9–15.

Shanas, E., & Maddox, G. L. (1976). Aging, health, and the organization of health resources. In R. H. Binstock & E. Shanas (Eds.), *Handbook of aging and the social sciences* (pp. 592–618). New York: Van Nostrand Reinhold.

Shanas, E., Townsend, P., Wedderbrun, D., Friis, H., Milhøj, P., & Stehouwer, J. (1968). *Old people in three industrial societies.* New York: Atherton.

Shepherd, A. A. M., Hewick, D. S., Moreland, T. A., & Stevenson, I. H.

(1977). Age as a determinant of sensitivity to warfarin. *British Journal of Clinical Pharmacology, 4,* 315–320.

Sherman, B. M., West, J. H., & Korenman, S. G. (1976). The menopausal transition: Analysis of LH, FSH, estradiol, and progesterone concentration during menstrual cycles of older women. *Journal of Clinical Endocrinology and Metabolism, 42,* 629.

Sherwood, S. (Ed.) (1975). *Long-term care: A handbook for researchers, planners, and providers.* New York: Spectrum.

Shock, N. W. (1970). Physiologic aspects of aging. *Journal of the American Dietetic Association, 56,* 491–496.

Shock, N. W. (1977). Systems integration. In C. Finch & L. Hayflick (Eds.), *Handbook of the biology of aging* (pp. 639-665). New York: Van Nostrand Reinhold.

Sidney, K. H., & Shephard, R. J. (1977). Activity patterns of elderly men and women. *Journal of Gerontology, 32,* 25-32.

Siegler, L. C., & George, L. K. (in press). Sex differences in coping and perception of life events. *Journal of Geriatric Psychiatry.*

Silverman, P. R. (1974). *Helping each other in widowhood.* New York: Health Sciences.

Smith, D. C., Prentice, R., Thompson, D. J., & Herrmann, W. L. (1975). Association of exogenous estrogen and endometrial carcinoma. *New England Journal of Medicine, 293,* 1164-1167.

Smith, D. W., Bierman, E. L., & Robinson, N. M. (Eds.). (1978). *The biologic ages of man: From conception through old age* (2nd ed.). Philadelphia: Saunders.

Smith, E. V., Jr., Reddan, W., & Smith, P. E. (1981). Physical activity and calcium modalities for bone mineral increase in aged women. *Medicine and Science in Sports and Exercise, 13,* 60-64.

Smith, K. F., & Bengtson, V. L. (1979). Positive consequences of institutionalization: Solidarity between parents and their middle-aged children. *Gerontologist, 19,* 438–447.

Smith, L. (1983). *Meeting filial responsibility demands in middle age.* Unpublished Masters thesis, The Pennsylvania State University.

Smyer, M. A. (1980). The differential usage of services by impaired elderly. *Journal of Gerontology, 35,* 249-255.

Smyer, M. A., & Hofland, B. F. (1982). Divorce and family support in later life: Emerging concerns. *Journal of Family Issues, 3,* 61-77.

Snyder, D. (1979). Elderly poor: Effects of public transfers. *Journal of Minority Aging, 4,* 109-112.

Soberal-Perez v. Schweiker, 549 F. Supp. 1164 (E. D. New York, 1982).

Somerville, B. W. (1972). The influence of hormones upon migraine in women. *Medical Journal of Australia, 2,* (2, Spec. Supp.), 6–11.

Spaspoff, R. A., Kraus, A. S., Beattie, E. J., Holden, D. E. W., Lawson, J. S., Rodenberg, M., & Woodcock, G. M. (1978). A longitudinal study of elderly residents of long-stay institutions: I. Early response to institutional care. *Gerontologist, 18,* 281-292.

Special Committee on Aging. (1977). *Developments in aging, 1976.* Report of the Special Committee on Aging, U.S. Congress, Senate, No. 95-83. Washington, DC: U.S. Government Printing Office.

Spencer, H., Kramer, L., Norris, C., & Osis, D. (1974). Studies of calcium requirements in man. *Federation Proceedings, 33,* 714.

Spencer, H., Kramer, L., & Osis, D. (1982). Factors contributing to calcium loss in aging. *American Journal of Clinical Nutrition, 36,* (4, Suppl.), 776–787.

Spitzer, R. L., Endicott, J., & Robins, E. (1978). Research Diagnostic Criteria: Rational and reliability. *Archives of General Psychiatry, 35,* 773–782.

Streib, G. F. (1975). Mechanism for changes viewed in a sociological context. In P. B. Bart (Ed.), *No longer young: The older woman in America: Proceedings of the 26th Conference on Aging, 1973.* Institute of Gerontology, University of Michigan-Wayne State University.

Studd, J. W. W. (1979). The climacteric syndrome. In P. A. van Keep, D. M. Serr, & R. B. Greenblatt (Eds.), *Female and male climacteric* (pp. 23ff.). Lancaster, England: MTP Press.

Sullivan, D. M., Wood, T. R., & Griffen, W. O., Jr. (1982). Biliary tract surgery in the elderly. *American Journal of Surgery, 143,* 218–220.

Suominen, H., Heikkinen, E., & Parkatti, T. (1977). Effects of eight weeks' physical training on muscle and connective tissues on the M. Vastus Lateralis in 69-year-old men and women. *Journal of Gerontology, 32,* 33–37.

Talley, T., & Kaplan, J. (1956, December). The negro aged. *Newsletter,* Gerontological Society, 3.

Tingwald, G. R., & Cooperman, M. (1982). Inguinal and femoral hernia repair in geriatric patients. *Surgery, Gynecology, and Obstetrics, 154,* 704–706.

Tinsley, B. R., & Parke, R. D. (in press). Grandparents as support and socialization agents. In M. Lewis (Ed.), *Beyond the dyad.* New York: Plenum.

Tobin, S. S., & Kulys, R. (1980). The family and services. In C. Eisdorfer (Ed.), *Annual review of gerontology and geriatrics* (Vol. 1, pp. 370–399). New York: Springer.

Tobin, S. S., & Lieberman, M. A. (1976). *Last home for the aged: Critical implications of institutionalization.* San Francisco: Jossey-Bass.

Tobis, J. S. (1982). The hospitalized elderly. *Journal of the American Medical Association, 248,* 874.

Torrey, B. B. (1982). The lengthening of retirement. In M. W. Riley, R. P. Abeles, & M. S. Teitelbaum (Eds.), *Aging from birth to death: Sociotemporal perspectives* (Vol. 2, pp. 181–196). AAAS Selected Symposium 79. Boulder, CO: Westview.

Townsend, P. (1964). *The last refuge.* London: Routledge and Kegan Paul.

Treas, J., & VanHilst, A. (1976). Marriage and remarriage rates among older Americans. *Gerontologist, 16,* 132–136.

Treiman, R. L., Levine, K. A., Cohen, J. L., Cossmann, D. V., Foran, R. F.,

& Levin, P. M. (1982). Aneurysmectomy in the octogenerian. *American Journal of Surgery, 144,* 194–197.

Troll, L. E., & Bengtson, V. L. (1979). Generations in the family. In W. R. Burr, R. Hill, F. I. Nye, & I. L. Reiss (Eds.), *Contemporary theories about the family* (Vol. 1, pp. 127–161). New York: The Free Press.

Troll, L. E., Miller, S. J., & Atchley, R. C. (Eds.). (1979). *Families in later life.* Belmont, CA: Wadsworth.

Tsai, S. P., Lee, E. S., & Hardy, R. J. (1978). The effects of a reduction in leading causes of death: Potential gains in life expectancy. *American Journal of Public Health, 68,* 966–971.

Turner, J. H. (1978). *The structure of sociological theory.* Homewood, IL: Dorsey.

Uhlenberg, P. (1979). Older woman: The growing challenge to design constructive roles. *Gerontologist, 19,* 236–241.

Uhlenberg, P. (1980). Death and the family. *Journal of Family History, 5,* 313–320.

Uhlenberg, P., & Myers, M. A. P. (1981). Divorce and the elderly. *Gerontologist, 21,* 276–282.

U.S. Department of Commerce, Bureau of the Census. (1973). *Census Population: 1970.* Subject reports. Final report PC(2)-4E persons in institutions and other group quarters. Washington, DC: U.S. Government Printing Office.

U.S. Department of Commerce, Bureau of the Census. (1977a). Projections of the population of the United States: 177 to 2050. *Current Population Reports, Series P-25, No. 704.* Washington, DC: U.S. Government Printing Office.

U.S. Department of Commerce, Bureau of the Census. (1977b). *Social indicators 1976: Selected data on social conditions and trends in the United States.* Washington, DC: U.S. Government Printing Office.

U.S. Department of Commerce, Bureau of the Census. (1982a). Money income of households, families, and persons in the United States: 1980. *Current Population Reports. Series P-60, No. 917.* Washington, DC: U.S. Government Printing Office.

U.S. Department of Commerce, Bureau of the Census. (1982b). Preliminary estimates of the population of the United States by age, sex, and race: 1970 to 1981. *Current Population Reports. Series P-5, No. 132.* Washington, DC: U.S. Government Printing Office.

U.S. Department of Health and Human Services. (1980). *Promoting health/ Preventing disease—Objectives for the nation.* Washington, DC: Author.

U.S. Department of Health and Human Services. (1981). *1981 White House Conference on Aging: Report of the mini-conference on older women.* Washington, DC: Author.

U.S. Department of Health, Education, and Welfare. (1969). Marital status and living arrangements before admission to nursing and personal care homes, United States, May-June, 1964. *Vital and Health Statistics.*

(DHEW Publication No. PHS 1000). *Series 12,* No. 12. Washington, DC: U.S. Government Printing Office.

U.S. Department of Health, Education, and Welfare; Office of the Assistant Secretary of Health. (1979). *Healthy people. The Surgeon General's report on health promotion and disease prevention.* (DHEW Publication No. PHS 79-55071). Washington, DC: U.S. Government Printing Office.

U.S. Department of Health, Education, and Welfare; Human Services and Mental Health Administration, Center for Disease Control. (1972). *Ten-state nutrition survey, 1968-1970.* (DHEW Publication No. HSM 72-8130-8134). Washington, DC: U.S. Government Printing Office.

U.S. Department of Health, Education, and Welfare. (1974). *Preliminary findings of the first health and nutrition survey, U.S. 1971-1972: Dietary intake and biochemical findings.* (DHEW Publication No. HRA 74-1219-1). Washington, DC: U.S. Government Printing Office.

U.S. Department of Health, Education, and Welfare, Administration on Aging. (1975-1979). *Facts about older Americans.* (Annual Series). Washington, DC: Superintendent of Documents, U.S. Government Printing Office.

U.S. Department of Health, Education, and Welfare, Administration on Aging. (1976). *Elderly widows. Statistical Memo No. 33.* Washington, DC: U.S. Government Printing Office.

U.S. Department of Health, Education, and Welfare. (1979a). *Healthy people. The Surgeon General's report on health promotion and disease prevention 1979.* (DHEW Publication No. PHS 79-55071A). Washington, DC: U.S. Government Printing Office.

U.S. Department of Health, Education, and Welfare. (1979b). *The older woman: Continuities and discontinuities, Report of the National Institute on Aging and the National Institute of Mental Health Workshop. September, 14-16, 1978.* (DHEW Publication No. NIH 79-1897). Washington, DC: U.S. Government Printing Office.

U.S. Department of Health, Education, and Welfare, Federal Council on the Aging. (1980). *Mental health and the elderly: Recommendations for actions.* (DHEW Publication No. OHDS 80-20960). Washington, DC: U.S. Government Printing Office.

U.S. Department of Housing and Urban Development. (1973). *Older Americans: Facts about incomes and housing.* Washington, DC: U.S. Government Printing Office.

Utian, W. H. (1975). Definitive symptoms of post menopause—incorporating use of vaginal parabasal index. In P. A. van Keep & C. Lauritzen (Eds.), *Frontiers of hormone research* (Vol. 3, pp. 74-93). Basel: S. Karger.

Vallbona, C. (1982). Bodily responses to immobilization. In F. Kottke, G. K. Stillwell, & J. F. Lehmann (Eds.), *Krusen's handbook of physical medicine and rehabilitation* (3rd ed., pp. 963–976). Philadelphia: Saunders.

Van Coevering, V. G. R. (1973). *An exploratory study of middle-aged and older widows to investigate those variables which differentiate high and low life satisfaction.* Unpublished doctoral dissertation, Wayne State University, Detroit, MI.

Van Nostrand, J. F. (1981). The aged in nursing homes: Baseline data. *Research on Aging, 3,* 403–415.

Vaupel, J. W., Manton, K. G., & Stallard, E. (1979). The impact of heterogeneity in individual frailty on the dynamics of mortality. *Demography, 16,* 439–454.

Verbrugge, L. M. (1979). Female illness rates and illness behavior: Testing hypotheses about sex differences in health. *Women and Health, 4,* 61–79.

Verbrugge, L. M. (1980). Recent trends in sex mortality differentials in the United States. *Women and Health, 5,* 17–37.

Verbrugge, L. M. (1982a). Sex differentials in health. *Public Health Reports, 97,* 417–437.

Verbrugge, L. M. (1982b). Women and men: Mortality and health of older people. In M. W. Riley, B. B. Hess, & K. Bond (Eds.), *Aging in society: Selected reviews of recent research* (pp. 139–174). Hillsdale, NJ: L. Erlbaum.

Verbrugge, L. M. (1983a, April). *Longer life but worsening health? Trends in health and mortality of middle-aged and older persons.* Paper presented at the Population Association of America meetings, Pittsburgh.

Verbrugge, L. M. (1983b). The social roles of the sexes and their relative health and mortality. In A. Lopez & L. Ruzicka (Eds.), *Sex differentials in mortality: Trends, determinants, and consequences* (pp. 221–245). Canberra: Department of Demography, Australian National University.

Vestal, R. E. (1982). Pharmacology and aging. *Journal of the American Geriatrics Society, 30,* 191–200.

Vestal, R. E., Norns, A. H., Tobin, J. D., Cohen, B. H., Shock, N. W., & Andres, R. (1975). Antipyrine metabolism in man: Influence of age, alcohol, caffeine, and smoking. *Clinical Pharmacology and Therapeutics, 18,* 439–448.

Vestal, R. E., Wood, A. J. J., & Shand, D. G. (1979). Reduced beta-adrenoceptor sensitivity in the elderly. *Clinical Pharmacology and Therapeutics, 26,* 181–186.

Waldron, I. (1976). Why do women live longer than men? *Social Science and Medicine, 10,* 349–362.

Waldron, I. (1982). An analysis of causes of sex differences in mortality and morbidity. In W. R. Gove and G. R. Carpenter (Eds.), *The fundamental connection between nature and nurture: A review of the evidence* (pp. 69–116). Lexington, MA: D. C. Heath.

Wallace, S., & Whiting, B. (1976). Factors affecting drug binding in plasma of elderly patients. *British Journal of Clinical Pharmacology, 3,* 327–330.

Ward, R. A. (1979). The never-married in later life. *Journal of Gerontology, 34,* 861–869.

Warheit, G. J., Holzer, C. E., III, & Schwab, J. J. (1973). An analysis of social class and racial differences in depressive symptomatology: A community study. *Journal of Health and Social Behavior, 14,* 291–299.

Warshaw, G. A., Moore, J. T., Friedman, S. W., Currie, C. T., Kennie, D. C., Kane, W. J., & Mears, P. A. (1982). Functional disability in the hospitalized elderly. *Journal of the American Medical Association, 248,* 847–850.

Watson, W. H. (1975). The meaning of touch: Geriatric nursing. *Journal of Communication, 25,* 104–112.

Weissman, M. M. (1979). The myth of involutional melancholia. *Journal of the American Medical Association, 242,* 742–744.

Weissman, M. M., & Klerman, G. L. (1977). Sex differences and the epidemiology of depression. *Archives of General Psychiatry, 34,* 98–111.

Weissman, M. M., & Myers, J. K. (1980). Psychiatric disorders in a U.S. community, the application of Research Diagnostic Criteria to a resurveyed sample. *Acta Psychiatrica Scandinavica, 62,* 99–111.

Weissman, M. M., Myers, J. K., & Harding, P. S. (1978). Psychiatric disorders in a U.S. urban community: 1975–1976. *American Journal of Psychiatry, 135,* 459–462.

Welch, C. E. (1969). Surgery in the twilight years. *Bulletin, 23' Congres Societe Internationale de Chirurgie* (Buenos Aires), *September,* 302–396.

Welch, C. E., & Whittemore, W. S. (1954). Carcinoma of the rectum in a centenarian. *New England Journal of Medicine, 250,* 1041–1042.

Wilen, J. B. (1979). *Changing relationships among grandparents, parents, and their adult children.* Paper presented at the 32nd Annual Scientific Meeting of the Gerontological Society of America, Washington, DC. *Gerontologist, 19* (5, pt. II), 160 [Abstr.].

Wiley, J. A., & Camacho, T. C. (1980). Life-style and future health: Evidence from the Alameda County Study. *Preventive Medicine, 9,* 1–21.

Willis, S. L., & Baltes, P. B. (1980). Intelligence in adulthood and aging: Contemporary issues. In L. W. Poon (Ed.), *Aging in the 1980s: Psychological issues* (260–272). Washington, DC: American Psychological Association.

Wingard, D. L. (1982). The sex differential in mortality rates: Demographic and behavioral factors. *American Journal of Epidemiology, 115,* 205–216.

Wingard, D. L., Suarez, L., & Barrett-Connor, E. (1983). The sex differential in mortality from all causes and ischemic heart disease. *American Journal of Epidemiology, 117,* 165–172.

Winsborough, H. H. (1980). A demographic approach to the life cycle. In K. W. Back (Ed.), *Life course: Integrative theories and exemplary populations.* AAAS Selected Symposium No. 41, Boulder, CO: Westview.

Wirth, L. (1945). The problem of minority groups. In R. Linton (Ed.), *The science of man in the world crisis* (pp. 347–372). New York: Columbia University Press.

Wolanin, M. O., & Holloway, J. (1980). Relocation confusion: Intervention for prevention. In I. M. Burnside (Ed.), *Psychosocial nursing care of the aged* (2nd ed., pp. 181–194). New York: McGraw-Hill.

Wolanin, M. O., & Phillips, L. R. F. (1981). *Confusion: Prevention and care.* St. Louis: C. V. Mosby.

Wolinsky, F. D. (1980). *The sociology of health: Principles, professions, and issues.* Boston: Little, Brown.

Worcester, A. (1968). In M. B. Strauss (Ed.), *Familiar medical quotations.* Boston: Little Brown.

Young, M., & Willmott, P. (1962). *Family kinship in East London* (rev. ed.). Harmondworth: Penguin.

Ziel, M. K., Finkle, W. D. (1975). Increased risk of endometrial carcinoma among users of conjugated estrogens. *New England Journal of Medicine, 293,* 1167–1170.

Zimmer, M. J., Sullivan, C. A., & Richards, R. F. (1982). *Cases and materials on employment discrimination.* Boston: Little, Brown.

Zube, M. (1982). Changing behavior and outlook of aging men and women: Implications for marriage in the middle and late years. *Family Relations, 31,* 147–156.

Zung, W. W. K. (1965). A self-rating depression scale. *Archives of General Psychiatry, 12,* 63–70.

Zusman, J. (1967). Some explanations of the changing appearance of psychotic patients: Antecedents of the social breakdown syndrome concept. *International Journal of Psychiatry, 3,* 215–237.

Index